Alarm Bells
in Medicine

**Danger Symptoms
in Medicine, Surgery
and Clinical Specialties**

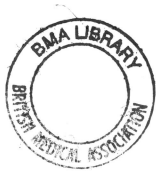

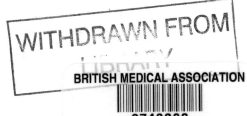

Alarm Bells in Medicine

Danger Symptoms in Medicine, Surgery and Clinical Specialties

Nadeem Ali

Specialist Registrar
Royal Victoria Infirmary, Newcastle-upon-Tyne

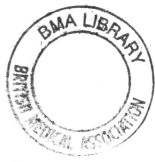

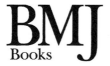 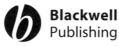

BMJ Books

Blackwell Publishing

© 2005 by Blackwell Publishing Ltd
BMJ Books is an imprint of the BMJ Publishing Group Limited,
used under licence

Blackwell Publishing, Inc., 350 Main Street, Malden, Massachusetts
    02148-5020, USA
Blackwell Publishing Ltd, 9600 Garsington Road, Oxford OX4 2DQ, UK
Blackwell Publishing Asia Pty Ltd, 550 Swanston Street, Carlton, Victoria
    3053, Australia

First published 2005

3 2007

Library of Congress Cataloging-in-Publication Data
Alarm bells in medicine : danger symptoms in medicine, surgery, and clinical
    specialties/[edited by] Nadeem Ali.
    p. ; cm.
    Includes index.
    ISBN: 978-0-7279-1819-2 (alk. paper : pbk.)
    1. Symptoms–Handbooks, manuals, etc. 2. Diagnosis, Differential–Handbooks,
manuals, etc. I. Ali, Nadeem. II. Title.
    Danger symptoms in medicine, surgery, and clinical specialties. [DNLM: 1. Diagnosis,
Differential–Handbooks. 2. Signs and Symptoms–Handbooks. 3. Medical History
Taking–methods–Handbooks. 4. Physical Examination–methods–Handbooks.
WB 39 A322 2005]
RC69.A445 2005
616.07′5–dc22

2005000980

ISBN: 978-0-7279-1819-2

A catalogue record for this title is available from the British Library

Set in 9.5/12pt Palatino
by SPI Publisher Services, Pondicherry, India
Printed and bound by TJ International Ltd, Padstow, Cornwall

Commissioning Editor: Mary Banks
Development Editor: Veronica Pock
Production Controller: Debbie Wyer

For further information on Blackwell Publishing, visit our website:
http://www.blackwellpublishing.com

The publisher's policy is to use permanent paper from mills that operate a sustainable
forestry policy, and which has been manufactured from pulp processed using acid-
free and elementary chlorine-free practices. Furthermore, the publisher ensures that
the text paper and cover board used have met acceptable environmental accreditation
standards.

Contents

List of contributors

Pertti Aarnio
Professor,
University of Turku,
Chief of the Department of Surgery,
Satakunta Central Hospital,
Pori, Finland

Mohan Adiseshiah
Consultant Vascular Surgeon,
UCL Hospitals,
London

Kosh Agarwal
Consultant Hepatologist,
Honorary Clinical Senior Lecturer,
Freeman Hospital,
Newcastle-upon-Tyne

Niruj Agrawal
Consultant Neuropsychiatrist and
 Honorary Senior Lecturer,
St George's Hospital Medical
 School, London

Farhan Ali
Clinical Research Fellow,
Writington Hospital, Wigan

Nadeem Ali
Specialist Registrar,
Royal Victoria Infirmary,
Newcastle-upon-Tyne

Robert Allan
Professor of Gastroenterology,
Queen Elizabeth Hospital,
Birmingham

Kamal Al-Shoumer
Associate Professor of Medicine,
Kuwait University,
Head of Division of Endocrinology
 and Metabolic Medicine,
Mubarak Al-Kabeer Teaching
 Hospital, Kuwait

Simon Barton
Clinical Director,
Department of HIV and GU
 Medicine,
Chelsea and Westminster Hospital,
London

Chandrima Biswas
Specialist Registrar,
Chelsea and Westminster Hospital,
London

Bernard Bochner
Urologic Surgeon,
Memorial Sloan-Kettering Cancer
 Center,
New York, USA

Jonathon Bodansky
Consultant Physician,
Senior Clinical Lecturer,
Clinical Director for Diabetes and
 Endocrinology,
Leeds Teaching Hospitals NHS
 Trust

Stana Bojanic
Specialist Registrar,
The Radcliffe Infirmary, Oxford

John Bradley
Consultant Nephrologist and Clinical Director of Renal Services,
Addenbrooke's Hospital,
Cambridge

Javier Carbone
Clinical Immunologist,
Gregorio Marañon Hospital,
Madrid

Cris Constantinescu
Professor and Head of Division of
Clinical Neurology,
University Hospital,
Nottingham

Christina Cotzias
Specialist Registrar,
Chelsea and Westminster Hospital,
London

Jeremy Crew
Consultant Urologist,
The Churchill Hospital,
Oxford

Mark Davenport
Consultant Paediatric Surgeon and
Reader,
King's College, London

Jill Dietz
Assistant Professor of Surgery,
Washington University School of
Medicine, USA

Adrian Drake-Lee
Consultant ENT Surgeon,
Queen Elizabeth Hospital,
Birmingham

Ahmed El-Gamel
Consultant Cardiothoracic Surgeon,
King's College Hospital,
London

Paul Emery
Professor and Head of the
Academic Unit of Musculoskeletal
Disease,
Leeds Teaching Hospitals NHS
Trust

Sadaf Farooqi
Research Fellow,
Addenbrooke's Hospital,
Cambridge

Martin Noel FitzGibbon
Consultant Gynaecologist,
Wordsley Hospital,
Stourbridge

Martha Ford-Adams
Consultant Paediatrician,
King's College Hospital,
London

Adele Francis
Consultant Breast Surgeon,
Queen Elizabeth Hospital,
Birmingham

Scott Fraser
Consultant Ophthalmologist,
Sunderland Eye Infirmary

Andrew Fry
Specialist Registrar,
Addenbrooke's Hospital,
Cambridge

Gennaro Galizia
Associate Professor of Surgery,
Second University of Naples,
Italy

Jeremy George
Consultant in Respiratory
Medicine,
UCL Hospitals,
London

Michael Griffin
Professor of Gastrointestinal
   Surgery,
University of Newcastle-upon-Tyne

Philip Griffiths
Senior Lecturer and Consultant
   Ophthalmologist,
Royal Victoria Infirmary,
Newcastle-upon-Tyne

Stein Erik Haugen
Head of Paediatric Surgery,
St. Olav's University Hospital,
Trondheim, Norway

Nigel Hall
Consultant Colorectal Surgeon,
Addenbrooke's Hospital,
Cambridge

Nick Hayes
Consultant Surgeon,
Royal Victoria Infirmary,
Newcastle-upon-Tyne

Peter Hayes
Professor of Hepatology,
Liver Unit,
Royal Infirmary, Edinburgh

Mike Hayton
Consultant Orthopaedic Surgeon,
Writington Hospital, Wigan

Richard Hillman
Senior Lecturer,
Sexually Transmitted Infections
   Research Centre,
University of Sydney, Australia

Steven Hirsch
Professor of Psychiatry and Head
   of Teaching Governance,
West London Mental Health Trust,
Charing Cross Hospital,
London

Sue Hobbins
Consultant Paediatrician,
Princess Royal University Hospital,
Farnborough

Shervanthi Homer-Vanniasinkam
Professor of Vascular Surgery,
Leeds General Infirmary

Graham Jackson
Consultant Haematologist,
Royal Victoria Infirmary,
Newcastle-upon-Tyne

Robin Jones
Specialist Registrar,
Royal Marsden Hospital,
London

Rose Anne Kenny
Professor of Cardiovascular
   Medicine,
Consultant in Geriatric Medicine,
Royal Victoria Infirmary,
Newcastle-upon-Tyne

Richard Kerr
Consultant Neurosurgeon,
The Radcliffe Infirmary,
Oxford

Patrick Kesteven
Consultant Haematologist,
Freeman Hospital,
Newcastle-upon-Tyne

John Langdon
Emeritus Professor,
Formerly Head of Oral and
   Maxillofacial Surgery,
King's College, London

Andrew Larner
Consultant Neurologist,
Walton Centre for Neurology and
   Neurosurgery, Liverpool

Gregory Lip
Professor of Cardiovascular
  Medicine,
City Hospital,
Birmingham

Paul Manson
Professor and Chief of Plastic
  Surgery,
Johns Hopkins Hospital,
Baltimore, USA

Andrew McLaren
Clinical Research Associate,
Newcastle General Hospital

Gary Miller
Chief of Orthopaedic Surgery
  Service,
Veteran Affairs Medical Center,
Associate Professor,
Washington University School of
  Medicine in St Louis, USA

Chas Newstead
Consultant Renal Physician,
St James's Hospital,
Leeds

Graham Niepel
Research Fellow,
University Hospital,
Nottingham

Robert Ord
Professor and Chairman,
Department of Oral and
  Maxillofacial Surgery,
University of Maryland,
Baltimore, USA

Sarah Pape
Consultant Plastic Surgeon and
  Director of Northern Regional
  Burns Network,
Royal Victoria Infirmary,
Newcastle-upon-Tyne

Petros Perros
Consultant Endocrinologist,
Freeman Hospital,
Newcastle-upon-Tyne

John Plevris
Senior Lecturer and Consultant
  Gastroenterologist,
Royal Infirmary of Edinburgh

Mark Roberts
Consultant Gynaecologist,
Royal Victoria Infirmary,
Newcastle-upon-Tyne

Laurence Rubenstein
Professor of Medicine,
UCLA,
Chief of Division of Geriatric
  Medicine,
Greater Los Angeles VA Medical
  Center,
USA

Robert Sanders
Rosalind Franklin University of
  Medicine and Science,
Chicago, USA

Lori Siegel
Professor and Chief of Division of
  Rheumatology,
Rosalind Franklin University of
  Medicine and Science,
Chicago, USA

Navin Singh
Assistant Professor,
Johns Hopkins Hospital,
Baltimore,
USA

Ian Smith
Professor of Cancer Medicine and
  Head of Breast Unit,
Royal Marsden Hospital,
London

Gavin Spickett
Consultant Immunologist,
Royal Victoria Infirmary,
Newcastle-upon-Tyne

Gerard Stansby
Professor of Vascular Surgery,
University of Newcastle-upon-Tyne

Richard Staughton
Consultant Dermatologist,
Chelsea and Westminster
   Hospital,
London

Philip Steer
Professor and Head of Department
   of Maternal and Fetal Medicine,
Imperial College,
Chelsea and Westminster
   Hospital,
London

Chris Stenton
Consultant in Respiratory
   Medicine,
Royal Victoria Infirmary,
Newcastle-upon-Tyne

David Talbot
Consultant Transplant Surgeon,
Freeman Hospital,
Newcastle-upon-Tyne

Muzahir Tayebjee
Research Fellow,
City Hospital, Birmingham

Emma Topham
Specialist Registrar,
Chelsea and Westminster Hospital,
London

Jonathan Wasserberg
Consultant Neurosurgeon,
Queen Elizabeth Hospital,
Birmingham

Peter-John Wormald
Professor of Otolaryngology,
University of Adelaide,
Australia

Guy Wynne-Jones
Specialist Registrar,
Queen Elizabeth Hospital,
Birmingham

Introduction

As a clinical student, I never felt I gained much from didactic teaching. The greatest exception to this was a lesson taught by Peter Ellis, Consultant ENT Surgeon at Addenbrooke's hospital. He had the daunting prospect of taking an uninspired group of students for the whole afternoon in a small, stuffy lecture room. He made us take our seats, then, sitting on a table at the front, he announced, 'I am going to teach you something today that you are never going to forget. Any patient with hoarseness of the voice for 3 weeks has carcinoma of the larynx until proven otherwise. Right, off you go.' The lesson was over, and he proved correct in his prediction that it would remain unfaded in our memories.

This lesson taught me several things. First, that a little knowledge retained is worth more than a lot forgotten. Second, that the primary knowledge in medicine is that which will save life or limb. Third, that certain symptoms should make your ears prick up, your neck hairs bristle and your heart pound, springing you into action. Symptoms such as this are what make up this book – they are 'alarm bells'.

Of course, every area of medicine, surgery and the clinical specialities has its own alarm bells, those crucial symptoms that, if missed, may lead to death or demise (of the patient and, increasingly, the doctor). These are the clinical pearls that slip out on the ward rounds and in the clinics of experienced doctors. This book is therefore a beachcombing exercise, gathering all these vital symptoms from every area of clinical practice, and depositing them in a single casket.

Symptoms, not signs, have been included. This is because every doctor, no matter how subspecialised, can be exposed to the full range of medical symptoms, just by virtue of the patient's speech. He is unlikely, however, to be presented with, or capable of eliciting, a comparable range of signs on examination. An ophthalmologist is unlikely to be adept at picking up splenomegaly, or a haematologist at detecting peripheral retinal neovascularisation – two signs of chronic myeloid leukaemia. However, both doctors can remember that, if a patient complains of generalised itch, he may be suffering from the condition.

The methodology of the book is as follows. For each clinical speciality, at least two experienced doctors suggested, independently, up to 10 alarm bells for their field. Whatever alarm bells were suggested by both specialists were assumed to be important and included in the final chapter. The remainder were assessed on their own merits to make the final list, with a maximum of ten. (Paediatrics, given its exceptionally broad range, was allowed 15.)

In some ways, this is an unfashionable book. It contains no evidence, no guidelines, no protocols, no references, even. It does, however, contain the combined clinical wisdom of over 70 experienced doctors from around the world, with their cumulative centuries of listening to patients.

Acknowledgement

I wish to express my thanks to my wife, Dr Sadia Mohiud-Din. Not only does she deserve the credit for the original idea, for contacting contributors, and for reviewing the text, but also for supporting me throughout. If she finds this book useful to her practice, I will be happy enough. Thanks are also due to Mary Banks, Commissioning Editor, and Veronica Pock, Development Editor, both pivotal in giving form to the concept. Finally, I record my appreciation of all the contributors who enthusiastically engaged in this novel venture, shared their clinical wisdom with generosity and humility, and taught me a lot.

DEDICATION

To Talat and Ghufran Ali, grandparents of Musa

Abbreviations

5-HIAA	5-hydroxyindoleacetic acid
AAA	abdominal aortic aneurysm
ABPA	allergic bronchopulmonary aspergillosis
ACAG	acute closed-angle glaucoma
ACE	angiotensin-converting enzyme
ACTH	adrenocorticotropic hormone
ADLs	activities of daily living
AF	atrial fibrillation
AIDS	acquired immunodeficiency syndrome
ALP	alkaline phosphatase
ANAs	anti-nuclear antibodies
ANCAs	antineutrophil cytoplasmic antibodies
APTT	activated partial thromboplastin time
BA	bile acid
BMI	body mass index
BP	blood pressure
CA125	cancer antigen 125
CHB	congenital heart block
CK	creatinine kinase
CMV	cytomegalovirus
COPD	chronic obstructive pulmonary disease
CPR	cardiopulmonary resuscitation
CRP	C-reactive protein
CSF	cerebrospinal fluid
CT	computed tomography
CXR	chest X-ray
DKA	diabetic ketoacidosis
DLB	dementia with Lewy bodies
DVLA	Driver and Vehicle Licensing Authority
DVT	deep venous thrombosis
ECG	electrocardiogram

EDH	extradural haematoma
ENT	ear, nose and throat
ESR	erythrocyte sedimentation rate
FBC	full blood count
FFP	fresh frozen plasma
FNA	fine-needle aspiration
FOB	faecal occult blood
GBS	Guillain-Barré syndrome
GCA	giant cell arteritis
GI	gastrointestinal
GP	general practitioner
HAE	hereditary angio-oedema
HIV	human immunodeficiency virus
HRT	hormone replacement therapy
HSV	herpes simplex virus
IADLs	instrumental activities of daily living
ICP	intracranial pressure
ICU	intensive care unit
IgE	immunoglobulin E
IgG	immunoglobulin G
IM	intramuscular
IV	intravenous
K	potassium
LFTs	liver function tests
LRTI	lower respiratory tract infection
MG	myasthenia gravis
MI	myocardial infarction
MRI	magnetic resonance imaging
Na	sodium
NSAIDs	non-steroidal anti-inflammatory drugs
PCOS	polycystic ovarian syndrome
PCR	polymerase chain reaction
PD	peritoneal dialysis
PE	pulmonary embolism
PID	pelvic inflammatory disease
PPIs	proton pump inhibitors
PPROM	preterm prelabour rupture of the membranes
SAH	subarachnoid haemorrhage
SBP	spontaneous bacterial peritonitis
SLE	systemic lupus erythematosus

SUFE	slipped upper femoral epiphysis
TB	tuberculosis
TED	thromboembolic deterrent
TFTs	thyroid function tests
TIA	transient ischaemic attack
U&E	urea and electrolytes (including creatinine)
URTI	upper respiratory tract infection
UTI	urinary tract infection
VQ	ventilation perfusion
βhCG	beta human chorionic gonadotropin
γGT	gamma-glutamyltransferase

NOTES ON REFERRAL

There is an explanatory paragraph for each Alarm Bell which includes instructions on what action should be taken. This usually involves referring to a specialist team. When the instruction is just to 'refer', it means non-urgently. When the term 'refer urgently' is used, it means: so that the patient is seen, at longest, within a two-week period. 'Refer immediately' means: pick up the phone and get the patient seen within hours.

Breast surgery

Adele Francis and Jill Dietz

1 A discrete breast lump does not need reviewing, it needs referring.

2 Breast lumps in young women probably are not cancer, but may be.

3 Do not ignore breast lumps in pregnant women: their relatively poor prognosis is due to delay in diagnosis.

4 Skin dimpling or retraction is usually caused by breast cancer.

5 All spontaneous nipple discharge (bloody or not) should be evaluated.

6 An inflamed breast may be an inflammatory carcinoma, not infection.

7 A complaint of a change in breast size or shape may signify malignancy.

8 Unilateral nipple inversion of recent onset may be caused by an underlying carcinoma.

9 An axillary mass could be breast cancer even with a normal breast examination.

10 Men also get breast cancer.

NOTES

1 Breast lump

Approximately one in ten patients with a discrete breast lump has cancer. Benign lumps are common but so are cancers, particularly in postmenopausal women. All lumps undergo triple assessment in the breast clinic: clinical examination, imaging and cytology or pathology. Clinical examination alone is not enough, as some cancers may be missed.

Action: Refer urgently to the breast unit.

2 Breast lumps in young women

Every breast unit in the country diagnoses patients with breast cancer in their twenties and thirties. A delay in referral can directly lead to a poor prognosis. Any young patient with signs or symptoms of breast cancer should not be reassured or reviewed, but referred.

Action: Refer urgently to the breast unit.

3 Breast lumps in pregnancy

There is significant evidence that, stage for stage, age for age, breast cancer diagnosed during pregnancy has the same prognosis as that diagnosed in non-pregnant women. The anecdotal poor outcome is due to the well-documented delay in diagnosis that occurs, both because of reluctance by the physician to refer and reluctance, once referred, to perform the appropriate diagnostic investigations. Breast lumps are not a normal side-effect of pregnancy.

Action: Refer urgently to the breast unit.

4 Skin dimpling and retraction

Skin dimpling and retraction rarely occur in the setting of benign breast disease. A malignancy or the surrounding reaction can cause retraction of Cooper's ligaments, which attach to the skin. In addition, cancer can involve skin directly. Often the patient has not noticed the underlying lump, and complains of the skin changes only.

Action: Refer urgently to the breast unit.

5 Nipple discharge

The diagnosis of pathologic nipple discharge is a clinical one. Bloody discharge is never normal. Ductal carcinoma must be suspected. In addition, spontaneous, unilateral discharge, which is serous or watery, can also be caused by intraductal pathology and warrants further investigation. While only 10% of pathologic nipple discharge cases are malignant, all spontaneous discharge should be evaluated.

Action: Refer urgently to the breast unit.

6 Inflamed breast

Breasts can go red and hard with infection (acute mastitis) and also with a rapidly progressing inflammatory breast cancer. The diagnosis can be made with time and response to antibiotics but much more quickly by urgent referral for triple assessment.

Action: Give appropriate antibiotics and refer urgently to the breast unit.

7 New breast asymmetry

Sometimes a woman or physician will notice a swelling or shrinking of one breast or flattening of the breast with arm movement and no evidence of a mass. Lobular cancers can be very infiltrative and yet might not produce a mass. Cancer or its fibrous reaction can cause retraction of Cooper's ligaments causing a shape change in the breast. Every breast exam should include visual inspection with the arms in various positions.

Action: Refer urgently to the breast clinic.

8 Nipple inversion

Many women have long-standing bilateral nipple inversion of many years' history and this is not suspicious. What should arouse suspicion is a unilateral inversion of recent onset, which may signal an underlying cancer.

Action: Refer urgently to the breast clinic.

9 Axillary mass

Breast cancer can present as an axillary mass from metastasis to the lymph nodes. Palpable axillary lymph nodes should generally be regarded as suspicious, particularly if large or hard. Often investigation reveals a breast mass or mammographic lesion. Occasionally, however, no abnormality can be found and an 'unknown primary' should be considered. Cat scratches or infected wounds of the arm or hand may also result in swollen lymph nodes. Infection will often cause tender lymph nodes or an erythematous lymphatic channel, and the primary site can often be identified. Other malignancies such as lymphoma can also present as an axillary mass.

Action: Examine lymph nodes elsewhere. Refer urgently to the breast unit.

10 Male breast cancer

Men rarely get breast cancer but when they do, it usually manifests itself as a painless lump under, or adjacent to, the nipple. The lump needs triple assessment to make the diagnosis.

Action: Refer urgently to the breast unit.

Cardiology

Muzahir Tayebjee and Gregory Lip

1. Sudden onset of tearing chest pain radiating to the back could be aortic dissection.
2. Sudden onset of syncope with palpitations and brisk recovery is typical of an arrhythmia.
3. Always include infective endocarditis in your differential for fever, weight loss and night sweats.
4. Central, crushing chest pain is MI until proved otherwise.
5. Exercise-induced chest pain needs rapid referral to exclude myocardial ischaemia.
6. Attacks of anxiety, flushing and palpitations in a hypertensive patient may signify a curable cause of hypertension.
7. Sudden onset of shortness of breath and pleuritic chest pain – think of pulmonary embolus.
8. Shortness of breath on walking or lying down could be heart failure.
9. Thyroid patients with palpitations may require anticoagulation to prevent stroke.
10. Investigate the heart in a young stroke (< 65 years old).

NOTES

1 Thoracic aorta dissection

If a patient presents with sudden onset, tearing chest pain radiating to the back, think of acute dissection of the thoracic aorta. Although rare, it carries a high mortality if untreated. Thrombolysis will kill in this condition, so always look for mediastinal widening on CXR before thrombolysing. The patient is usually very unwell, with nausea, sweating and pallor. If the spinal arteries are involved, there may be weakness; if the subclavian is involved, there may be radio-radial pulse delay. ST elevation may be seen on the ECG. Disorders of connective tissue, such as Marfan's syndrome, predispose. CT angiogram confirms the diagnosis, and emergency surgery may be required.

Action: Refer immediately to cardiology or cardiothoracic surgery (mortality increases by 2% every hour).

2 Arrhythmic syncope

History, especially from a witness, is crucial in the diagnosis of syncope. Cardiogenic syncope is likely when the onset is abrupt, dysrhythmia occurs, and recovery is quick when normal rhythm and circulation are restored. Syncope could be due to either a brady (e.g. asystole) or tachy (e.g. ventricular tachycardia) arrhythmia, and if palpitations are reported, their nature may provide a clue (slow, fast, regular or irregular). Structural heart disease (e.g. hypertrophic cardiomyopathy) or ischaemic heart disease often coexist with arrthymias and syncope. Remember that a broad complex tachycardia in a patient with ischaemic heart disease is ventricular tachycardia until proved otherwise.

Action: Take a detailed history about the event, cardiovascular risk factors, family and medication history. Perform a cardiovascular examination. Do an ECG. If the patient is haemodynamically compromised, unwell, or the ECG shows an arrhythmia, refer immediately; otherwise refer urgently to cardiology.

3 Infective endocarditis

Fever, weight loss and night sweats are features of infective endocarditis, lymphoma and tuberculosis. For all these conditions, the presentation is stealthy, and missing the diagnosis can prove disastrous. Risk factors for infective endocarditis include damaged native valves, prosthetic valves, permanent pacemakers and intravenous drug abuse. Untreated, infective endocarditis is fatal, resulting in haemodynamic compromise or systemic sepsis. Emboli from marantic vegetations can lodge anywhere within the circulation, resulting in stroke, peripheral limb ischaemia or gut infarction. The patient is often unwell and may have a new murmur.

Action: Take a detailed history and perform a full systematic examination. Listen for new murmurs. Refer immediately to the medical team.

4 Acute myocardial infarction

MI is a common medical emergency. Typically, patients present with central, crushing chest pain, radiating to the arms and jaws. Often these symptoms are accompanied by nausea, sweating, pallor and a sense of impending death. Younger patients may not have known risk factors.

Action: Give aspirin, and call 999. Do an ECG and thrombolyse immediately if there are no contraindications.

5 Chronic stable angina

Chest pain on exertion may indicate myocardial ischaemia due to coronary atherosclerosis. Patients at high risk include those with diabetes, hypertension, hyperlipidaemia, and those who smoke. Age is also an important risk factor.

Action: Take a detailed history and perform a cardiovascular examination, looking out for signs of valvular heart disease and heart failure. Do an ECG. Address risk factors, and commence aspirin and a beta blocker if there are no contraindications. Refer to the rapid access chest pain clinic.

6 Phaeochromocytoma

Phaeochromocytoma is a rare cause of secondary hypertension, but one that is often overlooked. It should be considered
in hypertensive patients who suffer from attacks of anxiety,
flushing and palpitations. Many patients report weight loss.
The anxiety symptoms are sometimes discounted as panic
attacks, but are due to sudden release of catecholamines from
the adrenal tumour. This may be precipitated by stress, or even
moving in bed. Removal of the adrenal tumour can cure the
hypertension, so early diagnosis can prevent hypertensive
complications.

Action: Send off a 24-h urine collection for catecholamines.
Refer urgently to a hypertension clinic.

7 Pulmonary embolism

The severity of a PE will reflect the degree of obstruction to the
pulmonary circulation. Presentation may range from a relatively well-looking patient to cardiovascular collapse. Tachypnoea is almost always present. Sudden onset of shortness of
breath with pleuritic chest pain is typical. Risk factors include
prolonged immobility, recent surgery, malignancy, central
venous cannulation, dehydration, clotting disorders (e.g. anticardiolipin syndrome in lupus) and oral contraception. There
may be a unilateral swollen leg pointing to a deep venous
thrombosis. Untreated, PE can be fatal or lead to severe
pulmonary hypertension.

Action: If arrested, start CPR. Give oxygen. Refer immediately
to medical admissions.

8 Heart failure

Heart failure can be caused by coronary artery and valvular
heart disease, and idiopathic cardiomyopathies. Characteristic
symptoms are shortness of breath on exertion, orthopnoea and
paroxysmal nocturnal dyspnoea. Patients may have deterior-
ated gradually or may present suddenly to the emergency department. Occasionally, treatment can restore cardiac function

to normal (e.g. mitral valve replacement) if the diagnosis is made early enough.

Action: In the acute setting, refer immediately to medical admissions. In other cases, refer urgently to cardiology.

9 Atrial fibrillation and thyroid disease

AF is the commonest arrhythmia, can occur as a complication of hyperthyroidism, and predisposes to stroke. Be alert, therefore, to thyroid patients who complain of palpitations. The risk of stroke increases with age and cardiovascular risk factors (e.g. diabetes, hypertension, valvular heart disease). Treatment involves managing the hyperthyroidism, controlling the ventricular rate and anticoagulating with warfarin.

Action: Ask patient to tap out rhythm (typically irregular) and identify other risk factors for stroke. Perform a full cardiovascular examination. A 12-lead ECG may identify the arrhythmia but ambulatory ECG monitoring may be required.

10 'Cardiogenic' stroke

A number of structural heart defects may predispose to stroke. These include atrial septal defects, congenital valvular defects, cardiomyopathy with ventricular thrombus and left atrial myxoma. Many of these can be easily treated (e.g. closure of an atrial septal defect). They must always be considered in a patient under 65 who presents with stroke.

Action: Refer for transthoracic or transoesophageal echocardiography.

Cardiothoracic surgery

Ahmed El-Gamel and Pertti Aarnio

1 A patient who is short of breath and tachycardic with extended neck veins – think of cardiac tamponade.

2 Syncope and dizziness could be due to aortic stenosis.

3 A tall, young patient with acute dyspnoea may have spontaneous pneumothorax.

4 In a young adult with hypertension, coarctation of the aorta must be excluded.

5 Consider underlying myocardial disease in all young patients with abnormal heart rhythms.

6 Chest pain after upper GI endoscopy – fear iatrogenic oesophageal perforation.

7 A patient with 'crackly' skin in the neck may have a ruptured bronchus or oesophagus.

8 Nocturnal cough or frequent chest infections in an old person could be due to pharyngeal pouch.

9 A car crash survivor who has sustained chest trauma may drop down dead at a later date.

10 Prolonged chest pain in a patient who has had recent open-heart surgery could be Dressler's syndrome.

NOTES

1 Cardiac tamponade

Cardiac tamponade carries a high mortality. It is caused by fluid accumulation in the pericardial space, which inhibits venous return, resulting in hypotension and cardiogenic shock. The fluid is either blood (trauma, surgery) or a large pericardial effusion (commonly malignant). The degree of cardiovascular compromise depends on the rate of fluid accumulation – small volumes may be fatal if the accumulation is acute. Acutely, the patient may be anxious, tachycardic, short of breath, with distended neck veins. Diagnosis depends on three cardinal features: falling blood pressure; rising jugular venous pressure; small, quiet heart. Emergency pericardial drainage is needed.

Action: Refer immediately to cardiothoracic surgery.

2 Aortic stenosis

Aortic valve stenosis may remain asymptomatic for years. During this time, hypertrophy normalises left ventricular wall stress. Eventually, symptoms appear as stenosis worsens and ventricular stress cannot be compensated for. The classic symptoms of aortic stenosis are angina, syncope and the symptoms of congestive heart failure. Most patients with moderate to severe aortic stenosis develop symptoms. Average survival after onset of angina is approximately 4 years; after syncope, 3 years; and after congestive heart failure, approximately 2 years. Congestive heart failure is the commonest cause of death, but some patients die suddenly. The classic examination finding is ejection systolic murmur over the aortic area.

Action: Arrange echocardiogram to confirm the diagnosis and refer to cardiology or cardiothoracic surgery. Avoid ACE inhibitors. Treat angina with beta blockers.

3 Spontaneous pneumothorax

Patients with spontaneous pneumothorax may develop dys-pnoea, pleuritic chest pain, hypoxia, arrhythmias, increased airway pressures or hypotension. In stable patients, the diag-nosis is suspected by absent breath sounds and is confirmed by CXR. With tension pneumothorax, respiratory distress is present, and the trachea is deviated away from the affected lung. This is a life-threatening emergency.

Action: For tension pneumothorax, immediately insert a large-bore needle (or thoracostomy tube) in the second anterior rib interspace in the mid-clavicular line. Apply closed suction until the patient is able to breathe spontaneously.

4 Aortic coarctation

Aortic coarctation in adults usually presents with upper-body hypertension typically in the second or third decade of life. Although these patients comprise a selected group that has survived beyond childhood, long-term complications can still occur. These include aneurysm formation of the aorta and the intercostal arteries. Other complications include premature cor-onary artery disease, left ventricular hypertrophy, endocarditis, and intracranial haemorrhage. Later in life, beyond 40 years, congestive heart failure may develop due to cardiomyopathy. Up to 40% of patients have associated bicuspid aortic valves that also may become stenotic and/or incompetent. CT or MRI may help in diagnosis.

Action: Refer to cardiothoracic surgery.

5 Myocardial disease

Arrhythmias in young patients require exclusion of underlying myocardial disease. Various arrhythmias can complicate myo-carditis, an acute inflammation of heart muscle. The patient may present with features similar to MI or with features of heart failure. AF is seen in some patients with cardiomyop-athies (obstructive and dilated). These patients are at risk of sudden death.

Action: Do ECG, CXR, echocardiography, and check viral serology and markers of connective tissue disease. Refer to cardiology.

6 Iatrogenic oesophageal perforation

Chest pain after upper GI endoscopy should raise suspicion about possible oesophageal perforation. The consequences are serious: contamination of perioesophageal spaces with corrosive digestive fluids and bacteria, leading to cellulitis and suppuration in the mediastinum. Pain, fever and dysphagia are the most frequent early features. Cervical crepitation may be palpated. CXR reveals mediastinal emphysema and pleural effusion with or without pneumothorax. X-ray imaging with opaque medium is required. Emergency surgery may be needed. Delay in treatment can be disastrous.

Action: If suspected, refer immediately back to the team who performed the endoscopy. Once diagnosis made, refer immediately to thoracic surgery.

7 Subcutaneous emphysema

Subcutaneous emphysema is air in the subcutaneous tissues. It can be diagnosed by palpating the skin for crepitation. Crackling is felt. Subcutaneous emphysema may complicate pneumothorax (treatment is as for the pneumothorax alone), but it may be due to bronchial rupture or oesophageal rupture, which may warrant emergency surgery. CXR confirms the subcutaneous emphysema and possible pneumothorax and pneumomediastinum.

Action: Refer immediately to thoracic surgery if there is pneumomediastinum.

8 Pharyngo-oesophageal diverticulum

Pharyngo-oesophageal diverticulum (pharyngeal pouch) usually occurs in elderly patients, more commonly in men. It is a progressive mucosal outpouching at the junction of the pharynx and the oesophagus. It may be asypmtomatic or cause dysphagia. In more advanced cases, collected food can regurgitate unpredictably, sometimes when turning at night. Recurrent aspiration can cause cough and pneumonia. At this stage, surgical excision is needed. Diagnostic endoscopy should be avoided due to the risk of inadvertent rupture during the procedure.

Action: Arrange barium swallow and refer for surgery.

9 Aortic transection

High-energy thoracic trauma is typified by the steering wheel injury in car crashes. In this scenario, injuries of the thoracic aorta may occur. Deceleration stresses can transect the aortic wall at the isthmus, immediately distal to the left subclavian artery. Most patients die immediately from exsanguination. In the few survivors, however, the periaortic tissues and pleura can produce a false aneurysm. This can then rupture into the pleural space at any time. Sudden death is therefore a continuing risk. As a result, the condition must be suspected on the basis of the history and excluded at the time of the injury.

Action: Do a CXR (widening of the mediastinum). Arrange aortography and refer urgently to cardiothoracic surgery.

10 Dressler's syndrome

The myopericardial inflammation associated with acute MI was first described by Dressler. This inflammation can also be caused by cardiotomy. In a patient who has had open-heart surgery, persistent chest pain may be due to Dressler's syndrome. Fever, friction rub and ECG changes suggestive of ischaemia may be present. Pericardial effusions may develop, sometimes causing haemodynamic compromise. Treatment is with NSAIDs – occasionally a course of steroids is needed.

Action: Check ECG, ESR (raised) and cardiac enzymes (normal). Arrange echocardiogram. Refer to cardiothoracic surgery or cardiology.

Care of the elderly

Rose Anne Kenny, Andrew McLaren and Laurence Rubenstein

1 In a patient who can no longer manage day-to-day tasks, search for underlying disease.

2 Dry cough may be the only symptom of heart failure in the elderly.

3 Falls could signify life-threatening arrhythmia.

4 Withdrawal can be a feature of delirium.

5 Depression is an old-age killer.

6 Fever and mental state changes – think of meningitis.

7 Clumsy hands may herald spinal cord compression.

8 Worsening breathlessness may be chronic pulmonary emboli.

9 Think of shingles before the skin lesions appear.

10 Acute confusion in a patient on neuroleptics or in a patient with Parkinson's disease could signal underlying Lewy body dementia.

NOTES

1 Functional impairment

Impaired function, as determined by inability to perform basic activities of daily living (ADLs) and instrumental ADLs (IADLs), is a sign of deterioration in many health conditions in older patients. ADLs include the basic functions of bathing, dressing, getting to the bathroom, transferring out of bed or chair, remaining continent and feeding oneself. IADLs include more advanced functions that enable a person to live independently: preparing meals, shopping, taking medications, managing finances, using a telephone, driving or using public transportation.

Action: Search for an underlying disease that may be contributing, such as a stroke, heart failure, pulmonary disease, dementing illness or infection.

2 Heart failure

Instead of dyspnoea, dry cough may be the presenting complaint of heart failure in older patients. Because of sedentary lifestyles, many older patients with heart failure do not experience progressive exertional dyspnoea. Furthermore, orthopnoea and paroxysmal nocturnal dyspnoea may not occur because of compensatory pulmonary vasculature changes and the common practice of older persons to sleep in a chair or recliner, rather than supine. Fatigue is also common. Diuretics may relieve symptoms.

Action: Examine for ankle swelling and listen for added heart sounds and chest crackles. Arrange echocardiogram, and refer to specialist services.

3 Cardiovascular syncope

While most falls in older people do not cause serious injury, 10–20% of them do, and falls often reflect an important acute or chronic systemic problem that needs to be elucidated. Unwitnessed falls, not due to trips or slips, in older persons who are cognitively normal may be due to cardiovascular syncope. Causes include hypotension and potentially life-threatening arrhythmias such as heart block and ventricular tachycardia. Such patients have amnesia for loss of consciousness. Two or more falls in a previously fit individual should raise suspicion.

Action: Check pulse, BP (including postural drop) and ECG. Refer to geriatric medicine or cardiology for further assessment.

4 Delirium

Delirium, or acute confusion or disorientation, is extremely common in acutely ill older people. It can stem from a large variety of acute conditions: cerebral hypoperfusion (from cardiac or cerebrovascular disease), metabolic abnormalities (e.g. electrolyte or hormonal imbalance), infection, medication (side-effects or withdrawal) or almost any serious acute illness. It is much more common in patients with underlying cognitive impairment or impaired vision or hearing. The presentation may be different in younger patients. There may be subtle symptoms of illusions or hallucinations and minimum apparent altered consciousness. Patients who are withdrawn with bedclothes over their heads are as likely to have delirium as those who are in a hyper alert, agitated state. Presentations of delirium are hyperactive in 15%, hypoactive in 20%, mixed in 50% and neither in 15%.

Action: Assess orientation. Look for evidence of chest infection or UTI and review drug history. Referral from the community depends on the level of social support and the ability to identify a treatable cause. If either is lacking, refer immediately to geriatric medicine.

5 Depression

Depression is a frequent and underdiagnosed killer among older adults. It occurs in 15–30% of older adults when looked for, but is identified much less frequently than this in usual clinical settings. As well as being the major risk factor for suicide, depression is often associated with worsening of medical illness and functional status through self-neglect. It should be routinely screened for in primary care settings through simple tests (e.g. Geriatric Depression Test), because when detected it can be usually improved with therapy.

Action: Screen older patients. Refer to old age psychiatry for further assessment.

6 Meningitis

The clinical features of meningitis in older people are subtler than in younger patients and the diagnosis is often overlooked. Acute mental state abnormalities with high fever and no other likely source of infection should raise concern about bacterial meningitis. Seizures are highly suspicious. Only half will have neck stiffness and meningeal signs and, because older people often have cervical spine disease and poor neck mobility, interpreting clinical signs can be difficult. Delay in diagnosis may partly explain the higher mortality rate in older compared to younger patients (55% versus 10%).

Action: Refer immediately to medical admissions or neurology.

7 Chronic spinal cord compression

Numbness and clumsiness in hands – think of chronic spinal cord compression. Cervical spondylosis is the most frequent cause of chronic cord compression in older people. Upper limb symptoms include numbness, clumsy hands, weakness and loss of dexterity. Lower limb symptoms include numbness, heaviness, weakness or a tendency to drag the limb.

Action: Refer all for acute neurological assessment.

8 Chronic pulmonary emboli

Patients with gradually worsening breathlessness may have chronic pulmonary emboli. In this situation, dyspnoea may be the only symptom, without pain or haemoptysis. Common risk factors include immobility, malignancy, recent surgery and hip fracture. Patients may develop signs of right-sided heart failure in addition to tachycardia and occasionally localised chest signs. There may be evidence of DVT.

Action: Refer immediately to medical admissions.

9. Herpes zoster

Herpes zoster (shingles) is easy to diagnose when skin lesions appear, but is frequently missed before that. Paraesthesia or dysaesthesia affecting a single dermatome is highly suggestive. Symptoms usually persist for several days up to a week before skin lesions appear. Oral antivirals (e.g. aciclovir) reduce the incidence of post-herpetic neuralgia at 1–3 months, and so can prevent significant morbidity.

Action: Treat with oral antivirals for 10 days.

10 Dementia with Lewy bodies (DLB)

Acute confusion in a patient with Parkinson's disease or in a patient on neuroleptics may be a feature of underlying DLB. DLB is one of a spectrum of movement disorder diagnoses. Parkinsonian features tend to present before cognitive impairment. Neuroleptic sensitivity is common in patients with DLB, and is not related to dose, duration of symptoms, or whether the agents are newer or not. As well as confusion, reactions may cause worsening Parkinsonism and irreversible cognitive decline. Severe reactions imply a poor prognosis. If it is necessary to prescribe neuroleptics to patients with possible DLB, close monitoring in a hospital setting is necessary, particularly when commencing treatment or changing doses.

Action: Stop neuroleptic treatment.

Dermatology

Emma Topham and Richard Staughton

1 Changing naevi need urgent referral to exclude melanoma.

2 A drug rash with blisters or erosions is life-threatening.

3 A febrile, young child with skin tenderness, flexural erythema and blisters may have staphylococcal scalded skin.

4 Generalised itching can be a marker of underlying systemic illness.

5 Purpuric rash or nodules on the lower legs may be presentation of systemic vasculitis.

6 Erythema involving 90% of the body surface can lead to death.

7 Urticaria with respiratory symptoms can be life-threatening.

8 Oral and genital mucous membrane ulcers may herald life-threatening disease.

9 Do not forget dermatomyositis in elderly patients with weakness, malaise and photosensitive rash.

10 Non-healing ulcers or crusty nodules may be malignant.

NOTES

1 Malignant melanoma

Malignant melanoma is the third most common malignancy diagnosed in those aged 15–39, and incidence is increasing. Survival is related to thickness at diagnosis, so early detection is vital. The ABCD rule can help clinically – A: asymmetry of lesion, B: irregular border, C: variation in colour, and D: diameter of lesion (> 6 mm is more suspicious). Do not forget subungual melanoma, which presents as longitudinal, pigmented streaks under the nail.

Action: Refer urgently to dermatology (2-week rule).

2 Toxic epidermal necrolysis

Toxic epidermal necrolysis is a life-threatening, acute condition characterised by widespread loss of epidermis due to a drug reaction. It has a mortality of 30%. The most important prognostic variables are how quickly the offending drug is identified and stopped, and the pre-existing comorbidity of the patient. Commonly implicated drugs are antibiotics, non-steroidal anti-inflammatory drugs (NSAIDs), anticonvulsants and antiretroviral drugs. Early features can include mild inflammation of eyelids, conjunctivae, mouth and genitalia, prior to skin tenderness, erythema, flaccid bullae and epidermal loss. A positive Nikolsky's sign (firm sliding pressure with a finger will separate normal looking epidermis from the dermis producing an erosion) and systemic upset are also found.

Action: Try to identify and withdraw the causative drugs. Refer immediately to dermatology.

3 Staphylococcal scalded skin

This is primarily seen in children under 5 and is caused by staphylococci that release an epidermolytic toxin. Important clinical clues are prominent denudation in areas of mechanical stress, easy disruption of the skin with firm rubbing and skin tenderness. Treatment requires IV antibiotics and supportive skin care.

Action: Refer immediately to paediatrics.

4 Generalised itch

Generalised itch in the absence of obvious skin signs should raise the possibility of underlying systemic disease. The differential diagnosis includes chronic renal failure, cholestasis, iron deficiency, polycythaemia vera, thyroid disease, malignancy and AIDS.

Action: Check FBC, U&E, LFTs, TFTs, serum electrophoresis, CXR, FOB. Refer to dermatology.

5 Systemic vasculitis

Cutaneous vasculitis may be the presenting feature of systemic vasculitis. Skin features may include purpuric papules, nodules and haemorrhagic bullae, commonly on the lower legs.

Action: Check BP and dipstick the urine. Refer urgently to dermatology or medicine for investigation of the underlying cause. Initial management is leg elevation, NSAID analgesia and bedrest.

6 Erythroderma

Erythroderma is defined as erythema affecting over 90% of body surface area. Possible causes are eczema, psoriasis and drug rashes. High-output cardiac failure, fluid and electrolyte imbalance and temperature dysregulation can result.

Action: Refer immediately to dermatology.

7 Urticaria

Weals or hives are a very common manifestation of urticaria. Angio-oedema is the deeper form of the condition, with soft tissue swelling that is usually perioral and periocular. Antihistamines are the mainstay of treatment. Danger symptoms include tongue or throat swelling, hoarseness and wheeze. These patients should carry an adrenaline auto-injector and wear a medic alert bracelet. An attempt to identify an underlying cause (foods, drugs, infection) should be made, although most cases are idiopathic.

Action: Supply an adrenaline auto-injector and refer to dermatology or allergy clinic.

8 Immunobullous skin disease

A group of rare skin diseases including pemphigus vulgaris, mucous membrane pemphigoid, erosive lichen planus and erythema multiforme can present with persistent and severe oral and genital ulceration with or without accompanying skin blisters and erosion. Diagnosis is made on the basis of skin biopsy for histology and immunofluorescence. Untreated, these conditions can progress to irreversible scarring and can be fatal.

Action: Refer urgently to dermatology.

9 Dermatomyositis

Dermatomyositis is an autoimmune, inflammatory condition affecting skin and muscle. Its associated weakness and malaise are gradual in onset and easy to miss. A photosensitive rash over face and hands can help alert to the diagnosis. Facial erythema, oedema and scaling, extending on to the V of the neck, and erythema of the hands may be all that is present, without the classical heliotrope erythema of the eyelids and erythematous papules on the hands.

Action: Check ESR, ANAs, CK. Refer to dermatology.

10 Squamous cell carcinoma

Non-healing ulcers and crusty nodules should be biopsied to exclude squamous cell carcinoma. Extra vigilance is required in transplant patients on long-term immunosuppression.

High-risk sites are the lip, ear, non-sun-exposed sites (penis, scrotum and anus) and areas of radiation or chronic ulceration.

Action: Refer urgently to dermatology (2-week rule).

Endocrinology

Petros Perros and Kamal Al-Shoumer

1 Any thyroid lump could be malignant.

2 A sore throat in a patient on antithyroid drugs could be due to agranulocytosis.

3 Pregnancy in a woman on thyroxine – detect undertreatment early.

4 Recurrent dizziness on standing and vomiting in a hyperpigmented patient suggests Addison's disease.

5 Worsening tiredness and malaise after starting thyroxine treatment may signify Addison's disease.

6 Sudden headache with collapse could be due to pituitary apoplexy.

7 Loss of vision to the side could be due to a pituitary tumour.

8 In a young patient with right-sided heart failure, episodes of flushing, diarrhoea, and wheeze suggest a neuroendocrine tumour.

9 New onset of hirsutism in middle-aged or older women is suspicious.

10 Prolonged numbness, tingling and muscle cramps after thyroid surgery – think of life-threatening hypocalcaemia.

NOTES

1 Thyroid cancer

Most thyroid lumps are benign, but around 5% are carcinomas. A palpable nodule is rarely malignant in a hyper- or hypo-thyroid patient, but is more worrying in a euthyroid patient. Features on history that suggest malignancy include being young (< 20 years) or old (> 70 years), male, previous external neck irradiation, previous thyroid cancer, recent changes in speaking, breathing or swallowing. Rapid growth is suspicious. In most cases, however, benign and malignant lumps cannot be distinguished on clinical grounds, and fine-needle aspiration (FNA) biopsy is needed. Ultrasound may complement, but not substitute for, FNA biopsy.

Action: Check TFTs. If normal, refer urgently to thyroid surgery or endocrinology. If abnormal, refer urgently to endocrinology.

2 Thionamide-induced agranulocytosis

In a patient on thionamide drugs (carbimazole, methimazole or propylthiouracil) for thyrotoxicosis, a sore throat associated with a fever and often mouth ulceration can signify agranulocytosis. The overall risk is low, highest in the first 3 months after initiation of treatment, but can occur at any time. Regular monitoring of FBC of patients on thionamide drugs is unnecessary, but education for recognising the early signs of agranulocytosis is mandatory.

Action: Do immediate FBC. Tell the patient to stop taking the drug until the result is available. Check the FBC result within a couple of hours. If agranulocytosis is confirmed, refer immediately to medical admissions. If the white count is normal, advise the patient to continue taking the tablets.

3 Pregnancy in a woman on thyroxine

It is possible that even mild under-replacement with thyroxine during the early stages of pregnancy can lead to subtle, permanent neurocognitive deficits in the offspring. Women on thyroxine need endocrinology advice and monitoring during pregnancy.

Action: Check TFTs in women on thyroxine when they declare a wish to conceive, or as soon as they have a positive pregnancy test. Refer urgently to endocrinology.

4 Addison's disease

Primary adrenal insufficiency (Addison's disease) is crucial to diagnose, and must be treated for life. Presentation is usually gradual: weakness, fatigue and anorexia are universal. There may be GI symptoms like nausea, vomiting, ill-defined abdominal pain or constipation. Symptoms of orthostatic hypotension, arthralgia, myalgia and salt craving may also be encountered. Hyperpigmentation, if not obvious, should be looked for in palmar creases and buccal mucosa. A first presentation as an acute adrenal crisis is rare, but may follow infection, trauma or surgery. Untreated, adrenal crisis is fatal. Suspect adrenal crisis in any hyperpigmented patient who develops prostration from vomiting and diarrhoea, with profound circulatory collapse and hypoglycaemia.

Action: Check U&E (K high, Na low, urea high), calcium (high), glucose (low), FBC (normocytic anaemia, neutrophils low, lymphocytes high), LFTs (abnormal). Refer urgently to endocrinology. In adrenal crisis, resuscitate with fluids (plasma expander then dextrose-saline), give parenteral glucocorticoids, and refer immediately to emergency department.

5 Thyroid hormone replacement and Addison's disease

Initiating thyroid hormone replacement in a patient with undiagnosed Addison's disease can cause deterioration of symptoms and in some cases an adrenal crisis. As a result, any patient recently started on thyroxine whose symptoms (e.g. tiredness and malaise) worsen needs exclusion of Addison's disease.

Action: Refer urgently to endocrinology. Do not increase the dose of thyroxine until investigated.

6 Pituitary apoplexy

Pituitary apoplexy is a rare, life-threatening event due to intra-pituitary haemorrhage in patients with large (often undiag-nosed) pituitary tumours. It typically presents with sudden, severe headache (like a subarachnoid) and collapse. More sub-tle presentations may be misdiagnosed as migraine. A low blood pressure (BP) (due to acute ACTH deficiency) and features of hypopituitarism are diagnostic clues. If the haem-orrhage continues to expand, diplopia, ophthalmoplegia and ptosis may result due to compression of cranial nerves cours-ing through the adjacent cavernous sinus. MRI and surgery are required.

Action: Refer immediately to medical admissions.

7 Pituitary tumour

Pituitary tumours may extend upwards, above the sella tur-sica, resulting in compression of the optic chiasm. The initial presentation may be loss of vision to the sides (bitemporal hemianopia), which, at first, may be noticed by the patient only on one side. Other possible pressure effects include headache, somnolence, epilepsy and CSF rhinorrhoea. Features of excess pituitary hormone secretion, or hypopituitarism, may be present.

Action: Examine visual fields to confrontation. Check for pos-tural hypotension. Refer immediately to neuroendocrinology.

8 Carcinoid tumour

Carcinoid tumours can be derived from foregut (bronchus, stomach and pancreas), midgut (small intestine and ascending colon) and hindgut (distal colon and rectum). Rarely, they may arise in the gonads. Carcinoid syndrome (flushing, secretory diarrhoea, bronchospasm, right-sided heart failure, pigmenta-tion, skin rashes) occurs in 10% of patients with carcinoid tumours. It results from the secretion of a variety of peptide products by the tumour. Diagnosis is based on the measurement of neuroendocrine markers (5-hydroxyindoleacetic acid (5-HIAA) in 24-h urine) and histology.

Action: Refer urgently to neuroendocrinology.

9 Hirsutism

Hirsutism is excessive facial and body hair, sufficient to cause concern to the patient. It is common in the general female population, and in most cases is due to polycystic ovarian syndrome (PCOS). Hirsutism occurring for the first time in middle life or later is suspicious. It could be due to adrenal carcinoma, androgen-producing tumours of the adrenals or ovaries, or Cushing's syndrome.

Action: Refer urgently to endocrinology.

10 Postsurgical hypocalcaemia

Hypocalcaemia following thyroid surgery is not uncommon. If persistent, however, it may indicate an insult to the parathyroid glands (directly or to their blood supply). Patients may complain of prolonged or severe numbness, tingling or muscle cramps. Physical signs of hypocalcaemia should be sought: facial twitch elicited by tapping over the zygomatic arch; forearm spasm induced by inflation of an upper-arm BP cuff for up to 3 min. If missed, there may be progression to tetany, seizures and arrhythmias. Urgent calcium replacement is needed.

Action: Immediately check corrected serum calcium level and discuss with thyroid surgery or endocrinology regarding management.

ENT

Adrian Drake-Lee and Peter-John Wormald

1 A hoarse voice for more than 6 weeks could be vocal cord carcinoma.

2 A slowly growing neck lump is suspicious, especially if over 2 cm.

3 An unwell, drooling child (or adult) with difficulty breathing could have imminent airway obstruction due to epiglottitis.

4 Stridor in a child with URTI – airway could be at risk.

5 Progressive, unilateral hearing loss may be acoustic neuroma.

6 Unilateral nasal obstruction with bloody discharge or paraesthesia – think of tumour.

7 Unilateral glue ear in an adult of Chinese origin is nasopharyngeal carcinoma until proved otherwise.

8 Ear pain on swallowing is highly suspicious for tumour.

9 A child who does not babble and fails to respond to sound may have a hearing problem.

10 A child with unilateral, smelly nasal discharge could have a foreign body in the nose.

NOTES

1 Squamous carcinoma of the vocal cord

A hoarse voice after an URTI is very common and in most cases does not indicate sinister pathology. However, hoarseness that persists after the URTI has resolved may indicate pathology of the vocal cord, such as carcinoma. The risk is greatest in smokers, especially over the age of 50. Hoarseness lasting 6 weeks needs endoscopic visualisation of the vocal cords.

Action: Refer urgently to ENT.

2 Neoplastic neck lumps

While many neck lumps represent benign lymph gland enlargement after infection, some are due to spread of cancer. If a lump is more than 2 cm, it is highly suggestive of tuberculosis or neoplasm. Cancerous lumps are usually firm, non-tender and may be tethered to surrounding structures. If the lump is associated with a chronic mouth ulcer, unilateral sore throat or persistent hoarseness, cancer is likely and needs to be excluded by fine-needle aspiration.

Action: Thoroughly examine the neck and the mouth. Refer urgently to ENT.

3 Epiglottitis

Infection of the supraglottis and epiglottis may result in progressive swelling of this region. It can occur even in patients immunised against *Haemophilus influenzae*. The patient (usually a child, but adults can also be affected) is unwell, sitting up, with a high fever. A very painful throat prevents swallowing, and drooling occurs. Stridor may be present. Intubation and emergency tracheostomy are sometimes needed. Non-specialists should not examine these patients – placing a spatula into the mouth may precipitate laryngeal spasm and an airway emergency.

Action: Do not examine the throat. Refer immediately to the emergency department for attention of the ENT surgeon.

4 Laryngotracheobronchitis

Children below the age of 4 years can develop progressive swelling of their subglottis (region below the vocal cords) and glottis (vocal cords) as a consequence of a viral URTI. This laryngeal swelling narrows the airway producing stridor, and can ultimately cause complete airway obstruction.

Action: Refer immediately to the emergency department. While awaiting transfer, place mother and child in a steam environment – run the hot taps/shower in the bathroom until the room fills with steam. Give an adrenaline nebuliser if available.

5 Acoustic neuroma

An acoustic neuroma is a benign schwannoma of the vestibular nerve that most often presents with unilateral, sensorineural hearing loss. As it grows, it compresses the auditory nerve resulting in hearing loss and tinnitus. Disruption of vestibular nerve function, or sometimes compression of the cerebellum, may cause dizziness. Patients may also complain of middle ear symptoms such as a feeling of pressure.

Action: Check corneal sensation (may be down). Examine the eardrum (normal). Refer urgently to ENT.

6 Nasal cavity tumours

Nasal obstruction is common and may result from hayfever, septal deviation, nasal polyposis or from chronic sinusitis. However, unilateral nasal obstruction associated with a blood-stained discharge, pain or altered facial sensation indicates a more sinister pathology from a nasal cavity tumour invading surrounding structures.

Action: Refer urgently to ENT.

7 Nasopharyngeal carcinoma

Nasopharyngeal carcinoma is particularly common in those of Chinese origin and occurs at an earlier age than most tumours.

A mass in the postnasal space may block the eustachian tube and result in unilateral, secretory otitis media (glue ear). As a result, any adult with unilateral hearing loss who is found to have glue ear should have the postnasal space examined and biopsied if necessary. These tumours can also cause unilateral nasal discharge.

Action: Refer urgently to ENT.

8 Upper aerodigestive tract neoplasm

A persistent history of ear pain on swallowing is highly suggestive of upper aerodigestive tract neoplasm and such a patient should be examined promptly by endoscopy.

Action: Refer urgently to ENT.

9 Childhood hearing loss

A child who does not babble and fails to respond to sound may have sensorineural hearing loss. Early detection and treatment is crucial to normal speech and language development.

Action: Refer for hearing assessment.

10 Nasal cavity foreign body

Young children stick things up their nose. If this goes un-noticed by an adult, an infection develops around the foreign body and the child presents with a unilateral nasal discharge. There is normally an anaerobic component to the infection, which causes a foul smell. Sedation or anaesthesia may be required for removal of deep objects.

Action: Refer urgently to the emergency department for attention of the ENT surgeon.

Gastroenterology and colorectal surgery

Robert Allan, John Plevris and Nigel Hall

1 Change in bowel habit – think of colorectal cancer.

2 Dark-red rectal bleeding could be caused by colorectal cancer or colitis.

3 Lethargy and shortness of breath may indicate anaemia due to GI pathology.

4 Weight loss and anorexia – think of abdominal malignancy.

5 Black stool indicates upper GI bleeding.

6 Sudden onset of severe abdominal pain may be a life-threatening perforation.

7 A severe attack of ulcerative colitis with fever and abdominal pain may be life-threatening.

8 A patient who is unwell soon after colorectal surgery has an anastomotic leak until proved otherwise.

9 Lethargy in a patient with an ileostomy may herald dehydration and renal failure.

10 Not all abdominal symptoms are caused by GI disease.

NOTES

1 Colorectal cancer

A persistent change in bowel habit for more than 6 weeks, especially to a looser or more frequent stool, is a high-risk symptom for colorectal cancer. Constipation is of lower risk and does not require urgent referral. Unlike many cancers, colorectal cancer is often curable when detected early. Investigation of the lower GI tract by barium enema or colonoscopy is required.

Action: Examine the abdomen, including digital rectal examination. Refer urgently to colorectal surgery.

2 Rectal bleeding

Rectal bleeding is very common but can be a sign of cancer or inflammatory bowel disease. Worrying features include dark-red bleeding, blood mixed with the stool or associated alteration in bowel habit. Flexible lower GI endoscopy is the investigation of choice. Bright-red blood with associated anal symptoms (lump, itchiness, pain) is usually from a benign cause.

Action: Examine the abdomen, including a digital rectal examination. Do FBC. Refer urgently to colorectal surgery.

3 Iron-deficiency anaemia

Sinister GI pathology may present insidiously through the effects of iron-deficiency anaemia. Symptoms include lethargy, malaise, breathlessness, palpitations and angina. Common causes of chronic GI bleeding are peptic ulcers, gastritis, gastric and colonic malignancy, colonic polyps, inflammatory bowel disease and colonic angiodysplasias. Sometimes (e.g. in right-sided colonic tumours) there may be no other symptoms to point to the diagnosis.

Action: Ask about medications (aspirin/NSAIDs, anticoagulation). Examine the abdomen, including digital rectal examination. Do FBC and FOB ($\times 3$). If iron-deficiency anaemia is proved, stop medications likely to cause blood loss and treat with oral iron. Refer to gastroenterology or colorectal surgery for investigation as appropriate. If there is severe anaemia, refer immediately for blood transfusion.

4 Abdominal malignancy

Weight loss and loss of appetite (anorexia) are common presentations of intra-abdominal malignancy. Additional alarm symptoms increase the suspicion. Stomach cancer should be suspected if the patient also reports change in taste, or feels full after small meals. Pancreatic cancer is suggested by epigastric pain that radiates to the back. Medical and psychiatric causes must also enter the differential. Abdominal ultrasound or CT may be needed to exclude malignancy.

Action: Examine the abdomen including digital rectal examination. Do FBC, U&E, ESR, LFTs and dipstick the urine. If there are still no clues, refer urgently to gastroenterology.

5 Upper GI bleed

Bleeding from the upper GI tract is common and leads to death in up to 10% of cases. It is characterised by vomiting of fresh or altered blood (haematemesis) and tar-black stool (melaena). Melaena often precedes haematemesis, and can occur without it. In oesophageal causes such as varices, however, haematemesis is usually the first sign. If upper GI bleeding is severe, fresh rectal bleeding can occur – in these cases, the patient will be shocked. Cardiovascular manifestations of blood loss such as fainting, postural hypotension or angina (in patients with ischaemic heart disease) may precede GI signs.

Action: Ask about risk factors (peptic ulcer disease, chronic liver disease, aspirin/NSAIDs, warfarin). Check pulse, BP. Examine the abdomen, including digital rectal examination, and test for blood in the stool. Take blood for FBC and cross-match. If patient is shocked (pulse > 100 and/or systolic BP < 100 mmHg), commence IV fluid resuscitation and refer immediately to emergency department. If patient is cardiovascularly stable, discuss with gastroenterologist on call, even if melaena has been present for several days.

6 Perforated viscus

Intestinal perforation presents with sudden onset of abdominal pain. The commonest sites are duodenum (from an ulcer) and sigmoid colon (from a perforated diverticulum). The site of initial pain is often an indicator of whether the perforation is upper or lower GI, but the pain rapidly spreads to involve the whole abdomen. Early recognition leading to rapid treatment will minimise the risk of death and the need for a stoma. There are usually no preceding symptoms. The classic sign on examination is 'board-like rigidity', but this may be absent in the elderly because of poor muscle bulk and tone. Erect CXR is essential to confirm the presence of free air under the diaphragm.

Action: Ask about peptic ulcer disease and ingestion of aspirin/ NSAIDs. Check pulse, BP. Examine the abdomen, looking especially for rebound, guarding and reduced bowel sounds. Commence IV fluid resuscitation. Refer immediately to surgery.

7 Acute, severe ulcerative colitis

Ulcerative colitis is characterised by acute attacks of diarrhoea with blood or mucus. If, in addition to this, a patient becomes unwell with fever, tachycardia, abdominal pain/tenderness, dramatic weight loss or dehydration, a severe attack must be suspected. The risk is death from colonic perforation. These patients should be admitted without delay. Anaemia, high white cell count, low albumin, and raised CRP confirm the clinical suspicion.

Action: Check pulse, BP, temperature. Assess for dehydration. Commence IV fluid resuscitation. Refer immediately to medical admissions.

8 Anastomotic leak

Any patient, who becomes unwell less than 14 days after an operation involving an anastomosis, should be considered to have had an anastomotic leak, until proved otherwise. Few patients have the classical presentation of pain, fever and abdominal tenderness. Leaks may present with vomiting, small bowel obstruction, isolated fever, shortness of breath, confusion, renal failure and even diarrhoea. A gastrograffin enema and/or CT should confirm the diagnosis.

Action: Refer immediately to colorectal surgery.

9 Acute dehydration

Patients with an ileostomy are less able to regulate fluid balance because they have lost the absorptive capacity of the colon. In the first few months following establishment of an ileostomy, dehydration can be a significant problem. Patients may not notice the symptoms, which can be quite vague. Extreme lethargy, high stomal output, low urine volumes and sometimes even fever can be the warning symptoms of dehydration leading to hypovolaemic renal failure. Admission is warranted for IV fluids and monitoring of renal function.

Action: Commence IV fluid resuscitation. Refer immediately to colorectal surgery.

10 Non-GI causes of abdominal symptoms

Abdominal symptoms and weight loss are common features of GI disease. Occasionally, however, the cause may be a metabolic or endocrine disorder such as diabetes mellitus, hyperthyroidism or Addison's disease. These will be missed unless specifically considered and excluded.

Action: Dipstick urine for glucose, do TFTs and a synacthen test where indicated.

Genitourinary medicine

Simon Barton and Richard Hillman

1 Altered vaginal discharge demands examination to exclude life-threatening causes (e.g. malignancy or retained tampon).

2 Change in discharge during pregnancy warrants investigation.

3 Vaginal discharge and pelvic tenderness – think of pelvic inflammatory disease.

4 Anogenital warts that do not respond to treatment may be neoplastic.

5 Anogenital ulcers that do not respond to treatment may be neoplastic.

6 Anogenital symptoms without detectable abnormalities – consider sexual assault.

7 Anogenital ulcer or widespread acute rash in a sexually active person – exclude syphilis.

8 A man with dysuria, urethral discharge and an acute arthritis has disseminated gonorrhoea until proved otherwise.

NOTES

1 Altered vaginal discharge

All women with altered vaginal discharge should have an accurate history that details the nature of the discharge (amount, colour, bloodstaining, odour). They should also have a careful vaginal examination, accompanied by a chaperone if requested. This is to exclude potentially life-threatening causes such as a retained foreign object (e.g. tampon), which can lead to toxic shock syndrome, or a cervical carcinoma. Furthermore, examination, and taking vaginal specimens for Gram stain and/or the measurement of vaginal pH, can be helpful in determining whether a discharge is due to bacterial vaginosis, trichomoniasis or candidiasis.

Action: Examine all women with altered vaginal discharge.

2 Sexually transmitted infection in pregnancy

While there is usually an increased vaginal discharge during pregnancy, it is important to consider infection, particularly if there has been a sudden change in appearance or smell. Sexually transmitted infections such as gonorrhoea, *Chlamydia* and bacterial vaginosis may contribute to the discharge. They may be associated with pregnancy loss and neonatal morbidity.

Action: Take a careful risk activity history and refer urgently to obstetrics.

3 Pelvic Inflammatory Disease

In women with vaginal discharge, as well as performing a speculum examination, it is recommended that a bimanual examination be undertaken in order to detect the presence of pelvic tenderness, which is a cardinal feature of PID. The risk of tubal infertility after one episode of PID is almost 20%, and this rises to over 50% after three episodes. There is evidence that the later the diagnosis is made, the greater the women's risk of the development of tubal infertility, and hence of subsequent pelvic pain and increased risk of ectopic pregnancy. Where PID is suspected, it is good practice to take appropriate microbiological investigations, and then to commence treatment while laboratory confirmation of a causative organism is awaited. Contact tracing to arrange screening and treatment of sexual partners is recommended.

Action: Treat suspected PID early.

4 Anogenital warts

Anogenital warts are extremely common and can usually be diagnosed clinically. They typically respond quickly to local treatment with creams, paints or physically ablative methods. If they do not respond, it is important to reconsider the diagnosis. Papular lesions in the genitals may be normal variants (e.g. coronal papillae), other dermatological phenomena (e.g. skin tags), other infectious causes (e.g. secondary syphilis), or neoplastic phenomena. A biopsy will often prevent unnecessary and inappropriate treatments, and allow the diagnosis of neoplastic conditions.

Action: Refer urgently to genitourinary medicine if not responding to treatment.

5 Anogenital ulcers

The most common causes of anogenital ulceration are infective, either due to herpes simplex virus (HSV) or *Treponema pallidum*. Non-infectious ulcers may be traumatic or due to dermatological causes such as lichen planus. However, whatever the initial clinical diagnosis, if a genital ulcer fails to heal after suitable treatment (for whatever diagnosis) for 1 month, it is recommended that the original diagnosis be reviewed and biopsy be considered to exclude malignancy.

Action: Refer urgently to genitourinary medicine if not responding to treatment.

6 Sexual assault

Sexual assault and abuse occur in all societies, but the victims often find it difficult to discuss matters. Patients may present with a variety of apparently unrelated anogenital symptoms, including atypical sensations, loss of libido, vaginismus, dyspareunia and erectile failure. Only a sensitive and thorough sexual history will reveal the true cause. It is important to screen for infections of the anogenital area and to exclude other pathology. Reassurance of the absence of disease may be helpful, but skilled and long-term support is commonly necessary.

Action: Refer urgently to genitourinary medicine and victim support services.

7 Syphilis

'The great mimicker' (as syphilis has been described) is on the increase with major outbreaks in several cities in Europe over the past 5 years. There is a significant synergy between the transmission of syphilis and HIV – in some outbreaks more than half the new cases of syphilis have been HIV-infected individuals. The manifestations of syphilis range from the minor to the hospitalising, but all practitioners should be aware that a new anogenital ulcer or a disseminated rash in a sexually active individual must be investigated with syphilis serology.

Action: Check syphilis serology.

8 Gonorrhoea

Disseminated gonorrhoea is a serious medical condition that requires prompt treatment. Clinically, it presents with a fever, malaise and an asymmetric, severe, destructive arthritis, which may involve a knee, ankle, wrist or even temporomandibular joint. One-third of patients develop a painful necrotic or papular rash. Very rarely, endocarditis or meningitis occurs in severe cases. Diagnosis is clinical and microbiological (blood cultures and synovial fluid cultures). A significant proportion of patients may present with the joint or skin symptoms in the absence of significant urogenital symptoms. The differential

diagnosis includes Reiter's syndrome, meningococcal septicaemia and rheumatic fever.

Action: Refer urgently to genitourinary medicine or rheumatology.

Gynaecology

Martin Noel FitzGibbon and Mark Roberts

1 Postmenopausal bleeding – think of endometrial cancer.

2 Unscheduled bleeding on HRT – think of endometrial cancer.

3 Postcoital bleeding could be cervical cancer, even with a 'normal' smear.

4 Pelvic discomfort, abdominal distention and dyspepsia could be symptoms of ovarian cancer.

5 Consider pregnancy, even if the possibility is denied.

6 Abdominal or pelvic pain in a woman of reproductive years – exclude ectopic pregnancy.

7 Abdominal pain, with a negative pregnancy test, could be ovarian cyst rupture.

8 'Being wet all the time' may signify a urogenital fistula.

9 Vulval ulceration or bleeding may be neoplasm.

10 Enlarging 'fibroids' – exclude cancer.

NOTES

1 Endometrial cancer

Unpredictable vaginal bleeding 12 months after the meno-pause may herald endometrial cancer. In women over 55, approximately 1 in 8 with postmenopausal bleeding have an underlying malignancy, two-thirds of which are endometrial. The other third comprises vulval, cervical, ovarian or bowel cancers. Prompt referral to a specialist for examination, trans-vaginal scan and biopsy are required. Early hysterectomy for endometrial cancers has a high cure rate.

Action: Refer urgently to gynaecology.

2 Endometrial cancer on HRT

Women taking HRT can develop endometrial cancer. Unsched-uled or irregular vaginal bleeding must not be presumed to be caused by the hormone replacement.

Action: Refer urgently to gynaecology.

3 Cervical cancer

Menstrual irregularities are common, but postcoital bleeding is suspicious – it could be due to cervical cancer. Regular (3–5-year) cervical cytology smears are recommended in all women aged 25–65 to screen for precancer changes, but a recent 'normal smear' does not exclude the possibility. Speculum examination and targeted biopsy are required for diagnosis. Early treatment of cervical cancers has a high cure rate.

Action: Perform a speculum examination. If cervix looks sus-picious, refer urgently to gynaecology, otherwise within 4–6 weeks.

4 Ovarian cancer

Ovarian cancer is often silent in its early stages, with presen-tation delayed until abdominal metastases have occurred.

However, in retrospect, women frequently give a history of pelvic discomfort for a considerable time before referral. This may have been labelled 'irritable bowel syndrome'. At a later stage, symptoms may be due to the mass, ascites and effect of widespread peritoneal metastases. Abdominal distension and dyspepsia may be reported. There may be personal or family history of associated breast or ovarian cancer in 5% – usually, however, there is no risk factor. A pelvic/abdominal mass and ascites may be found on examination. Transabdominal and transvaginal ultrasound scan is the first-line investigation. Early diagnosis may have no impact on survival but may improve quality of life.

Action: Consider pelvic ultrasound in cases of pelvic discomfort. If mass or ascites present, refer urgently to gynaecology.

5 Pregnancy

The medical care of all women of reproductive age must include the possibility of pregnancy. Never was the maxim 'If you don't consider it, you won't diagnose it' more true. Vehement denial of the possibility of pregnancy is not reliable. Urinary pregnancy testing is quick and accurate, and should be carried out if there is any doubt.

Action: Do a urinary pregnancy test.

6 Ectopic pregnancy

Ectopic pregnancy is common – rarely, it can be life-threatening. It must be considered in all females of reproductive age with pelvic or abdominal pain. There may be a history of pelvic infection, subfertility or assisted reproduction. Pain may be one-sided and associated with syncope or shoulder tip pain. Menstruation may be delayed or irregular, but do not be misled by a history of 'normal' periods in recent weeks, as vaginal bleeding and a tubal ectopic can coexist. Examination reveals pelvic tenderness and a closed cervical os. Catastrophic tubal rupture will cause massive intraperitoneal blood loss. Pregnancy tests must be carried out and, if positive, an ectopic must be excluded. Primary investigations include transvaginal scan and quantitative serum βhCG. Treatment includes salpingectomy or methotrexate therapy. Some cases will resolve spontaneously during monitoring.

Action: Do a urinary pregnancy test. If positive, refer immediately to gynaecology.

7 Ovarian cyst rupture

In a woman with lower abdominal pain, with a negative pregnancy test, gynaecological causes must still be considered. Ovarian/paraovarian cyst accident may present acutely because of cyst rupture, haemorrhage or torsion. Cysts may be physiological (e.g. corpus luteum), pathological such as ovarian tumour (e.g. teratoma or cystadenoma), ruptured/infected endometriotic cyst, or paraovarian (tubal). An ovarian mass may be difficult to palpate due to acute abdominal or pelvic tenderness. Ultrasound scan is the investigation of choice and serum CA125 should be estimated with ovarian tumours to determine risk of malignancy. Laparoscopy or laparotomy is considered depending on symptoms and scan findings. The cyst is normally removed but sometimes oophorectomy is required if it is non-viable.

Action: Refer urgently to gynaecology, immediately if symptoms are severe.

8 Urogenital fistula

If a woman complains of 'being wet all the time', consider a urogenital fistula and do not just attribute it to incontinence or UTI. Frequently, there is a history of recent surgery or radiation. Fistulae may run from the ureter or bladder to the vagina. GI fistulae may present as a smelly discharge, especially in elderly women.

Action: Refer urgently to gynaecology.

9 Vulval dysplasia

Vulval dysplasias are more common after the menopause. Skin changes may represent lichen sclerosis or intraepithelial neoplasia. Severe skin changes such as ulceration, contact bleeding and exophytic growth may indicate vulval cancer. All vulval abnormalities should be considered for local biopsy. Early surgical intervention can improve symptom control and prognosis.

Action: Refer to gynaecology, urgently if changes look suspicious.

10 Sarcomatous change in fibroids

Fibroids are almost always benign. However, they can undergo sarcomatous change, or may coexist with a developing ovarian mass. If the symptoms are changing, or the mass appears to be enlarging, additional pathology should be excluded.

Action: Refer urgently to gynaecology.

Haematology

Graham Jackson and Patrick Kesteven

1 Generalised itch may be the first hint of a myeloproliferative disorder.

2 Painful mouth ulcers could signal life-threatening neutropaenia.

3 'Pulled calf muscle' in a recent traveller could be a DVT.

4 Easy bruising of recent onset may indicate a platelet problem.

5 Constipation with back pain – think of myeloma.

6 An Afro-Caribbean child with an acute abdomen may have sickle cell crisis.

7 Tired and lethargic – check for anaemia.

8 Do not forget haematological malignancy as a cause for weight loss.

9 Night sweats could herald lymphoma.

10 Pain on drinking alcohol is a feature of Hodgkin's disease.

NOTES

1 Myeloproliferative disorders

The four myeloproliferative disorders (chronic myeloid leukae-mia, polycythaemia rubra vera, essential thrombocythaemia and myelofibrosis) are frequently indolent in their presentation. Characteristically they present with symptoms of tiredness and lethargy, or those associated with splenomegaly (abdominal pain) or hypermetabolism. However, the first symptom may be a generalised itch, commonly made worse by a hot bath.

Action: Check FBC.

2 Neutropaenia

Profound neutropaenia is often heralded by a rash of painful mouth ulcers. These may be small (2–4 mm) punched-out le-sions surrounded by an inflammatory erythematous halo, but with no pus. Such ulcers are routinely looked for in patients with haematological disorders or those on chemotherapy. However, profound neutropaenia may be an idiosyncratic re-sponse to a wide variety of other medications, or the first symptom in a rapidly evolving aplastic anaemia. Neutropaenic patients are prone to rapid onset of devastating and potentially lethal sepsis.

Action: Check FBC.

3 DVT

Around 5–10% of DVTs are precipitated by travel – whether long-haul flights or extended journeys by road. Traveller's thrombosis tends to affect younger and fitter patients than other forms of DVT and tends to involve patients who carry other risk factors for venous thrombosis. Unfortunately, most people are unaware of these other risks, which may be con-genital (thrombophilias) or acquired (malignancy, oestrogen-containing medications). Frequently symptoms will evolve when the patient is on holiday and will nearly always be misdiagnosed by the patient as a pulled muscle. Early diagnosis (including D-dimers and ultrasound) is crucial to prevent PE.

Action: Refer immediately. Most centres have a DVT assessment protocol in place.

4 Platelet dysfunction

Easy bruising nearly always indicates a problem with platelets. This may be due to insufficient numbers in the circulation, which in turn may be due to marrow failure, or more commonly, due to greatly increased rate of destruction in the circulation (e.g. idiopathic thrombocytopenic purpura or disseminated intravascular coagulation). Less commonly, easy bruising may reflect decreased platelet function, caused by drugs like aspirin or clopidogrel, or by inherited defects such as in von Willebrand's disease. Whatever the cause, loss of platelet function sufficient to cause spontaneous bruising means the patient is at risk of catastrophic haemorrhage.

Action: Check the platelet count. Refer urgently to haematology.

5 Myeloma

A frequent presentation of multiple myeloma is the combination of acute back pain and constipation. Both are common symptoms in the population and are usually benign. However, in myeloma, both vertebral collapse (back pain) and hypercalcaemia (constipation) are medical emergencies for which relatively simple manoeuvres are effective. Other features of myeloma are generalised bone pain, thirst, confusion, anaemia, weight loss and general malaise.

Action: Check serum calcium (high), and both blood and urine immunoglobulins for a paraprotein (20% of myeloma shows a paraprotein in the urine only). Arrange X-rays of the affected area looking for osteoporosis or classical lytic lesions.

6 Sickle cell crisis

An acute abdomen in an Afro-Caribbean child is likely to be due to the same causes of acute abdomen in any child.

However, it may be the result of a sickle cell crisis. If so, there may be a positive family history. Surgery on a child in a sickle crisis may precipitate bowel infarction.

Action: Request a haemoglobin electrophoresis, or whatever screening test the local laboratory offers.

7 Anaemia

Tiredness, fatigue and lethargy are common symptoms with many causes, of which anaemia is one of the most important. Anaemia is notoriously difficult to assess clinically but is simply and rapidly diagnosed with an FBC. Anaemia is not a final diagnosis and in all cases a cause should be sought.

Action: Check FBC. Patients with iron deficiency should be assessed for a source of blood loss.

8 Haematological malignancy

Unexplained weight loss is always a worrying symptom. It can be caused by most of the haematological malignancies, in particular, lymphomas and lymphoid malignancies. An FBC is part of the screen in unexplained weight loss.

Action: Check FBC. Examine lymph nodes, liver and spleen. Refer urgently to haematology or oncology.

9 Lymphoma

Hot flushes, feeling warm and heat intolerance are fairly common symptoms. Less common are night sweats, often described as 'drenching', with the patient needing to change bedding and nightwear frequently. Such severe sweats, associated with swollen nodes, weight loss and unexplained pyrexia, may herald the development of a lymphoma or a lymphoproliferative disorder.

Action: Examine lymph nodes, liver and spleen. Do a CXR to exclude significant mediastinal adenopathy. Refer urgently to haematology or oncology.

10 Hodgkin's disease

In some patients with Hodgkin's disease, alcohol induces painful swelling of affected lymph glands. In young adults with swollen nodes, 'B' symptoms (weight loss, fever, night sweats) and alcohol-induced nodal or chest pain, Hodgkin's disease should be considered. It may also present with a generalised itch without a rash.

Action: Examine lymph nodes. Do a CXR to exclude significant mediastinal adenopathy. Refer urgently to haematology or oncology.

Hepatology and hepatobiliary surgery

Peter Hayes, Kosh Agarwal and Gennaro Galizia

1 Abdominal distention in a patient with liver disease is worrying.

2 Clinical deterioration in a patient with ascites – think of spontaneous bacterial peritonitis.

3 Jaundice in the elderly is commonly malignant.

4 A patient with liver disease who has difficulty concentrating may have early encephalopathy.

5 Drowsiness in a patient with cirrhosis may have a life-threatening cause.

6 Pallor and tachycardia in a cirrhotic patient may signal a variceal bleed, even without haematemesis or melaena.

7 Bruising in a patient with liver disease could mean deteriorating liver function.

8 Generalised itch can be due to biliary obstruction, even in the absence of jaundice.

9 Intermittent right upper quadrant pain and fever with jaundice – suspect cholangitis.

10 Continuous abdominal pain and fever with retching – examine for guarding in the right upper quadrant.

NOTES

1 Ascites

Check for ascites in a patient with liver disease who complains of abdominal swelling. In cirrhosis the presence of ascites indicates decompensation or liver failure and its onset implies a 2-year survival of 50%. Alternatively, ascites can be due to portal vein involvement by hepatocellular carcinoma or hepatic vein obstruction (Budd–Chiari syndrome). Other aetiologies must not be overlooked: intra-abdominal malignancy (including gynaecological neoplasms), nephrotic syndrome, cardiac failure.

Action: Examine the abdomen (dullness on percussion, shifting dullness). Refer urgently to the liver unit.

2 Spontaneous bacterial peritonitis (SBP)

SBP is the infection of pre-existing ascitic fluid by translocation of organisms across the GI tract. It should be considered in any patient with ascites who starts to deteriorate. Although not universally present, suggestive features include diffuse abdominal pain, fever, dehydration, vomiting and diarrhoea. Diagnosis depends on paracentesis of ascitic fluid. Treatment involves IV broad-spectrum antibiotics. Prophylactic antibiotic treatment with norfloxacin is effective in preventing SBP.

Action: Refer immediately to medical admissions.

3 Painless jaundice in the elderly

Jaundice has many causes: haemolytic, hepatic and obstructive. Extrahepatic obstruction may be due to gallstones, malignancy (pancreas, bile duct, metastasis), pancreatitis or biliary stricture. The clinical features may include dark urine and bleached, chalky stool. In the elderly, jaundice commonly has a sinister, obstructive cause, such as pancreatic carcinoma or cholangiocarcinoma. It is frequently painless. Raised conjugated bilirubin, ALP, γGT, and bile salts fit with an obstructive cause. Ultrasound of the biliary tree is often diagnostic, but CT and MRI may be required. In the elderly, drugs are another common cause of jaundice (including obstructive biochemical picture).

Action: Check LFTs. Refer urgently to the liver unit.

4 Early hepatic encephalopathy

Hepatic encephalopathy results from altered amino acid metabolism due to liver failure. It may progress from precoma to coma. Its early features, however, are subtle and easy to miss. These include irritability, difficulty concentrating (which may impair skills such as driving) and constructional apraxia (e.g. inability to draw or copy a star). Be suspicious of patients with known liver disease who report mild cognitive deficits. Ideally, patients in jobs where they use machinery or drive should be monitored for minimal or occult hepatic encephalopathy using screening tests such as the number connection test.

Action: Refer urgently to the liver unit.

5 Drowsiness

Drowsiness in a patient with cirrhosis may be due to encephalopathy. If so, constipation, GI bleeding and sepsis are common precipitating factors. Other causes, however, must not be missed: head injury with intracranial bleeding and drugs.

Action: Refer immediately to medical admissions.

6 Bleeding varices

In a patient with cirrhosis and portal hypertension, vomiting blood (haematemesis) and passing dark stool (melaena) are well-recognised presentations for bleeding oesophageal varices. However, these features are not always present initially and hypotension, tachycardia and anaemia should raise the possibility of this serious complication.

Action: Try to detect melaena on rectal examination. Resuscitate with fluids. Refer immediately to the emergency department.

7 Coagulopathy

Patients who present with bruising and liver disease may have deteriorating liver function, their bruising being a manifestation of prolonged coagulopathy or decreased platelet count. This is often precipitated by the development of sepsis. A more uncommon cause may be vitamin K deficiency in patients who have cholestatic jaundice.

Action: Check FBC, clotting, LFTs. Refer urgently to the liver unit.

8 Pruritus

In biliary obstruction, serum levels of bile salts increase, which can cause generalised pruritus. In some cases, serum levels of bilirubin remain normal, so the patient is not clinically jaundiced. This is explained by the fact that bilirubin is actively secreted into the bile juice, whereas bile salts require a pressure gradient. As a result, when biliary pressure is slightly increased, secretion of bile salts is abolished (so serum levels rise) but bilirubin is still actively secreted (so serum levels do not rise). Other causes of generalised pruritus should also be considered (Hodgkin's disease, renal failure).

Action: Check LFTs (ALP and γGT will be raised even if bilirubin is normal). Refer for biliary ultrasound.

9 Ascending cholangitis

Cholangitis means infection of the biliary tract usually due to obstruction or stenosis. The obstruction can be in intrahepatic (many causes) or extrahepatic biliary ducts (mostly due to stones). The condition can be life-threatening. Patients experience attacks of right upper quadrant pain and jaundice, but in distinction to biliary colic, also suffer intermittent high fever. Shock may be present. Ultrasound and MRI are useful in diagnosis. Urgent drainage of the bile duct is required.

Action: Resuscitate with fluids. Keep nil by mouth. Refer immediately to surgical admissions.

10 Acute cholecystitis

Acute inflammation of an obstructed gall bladder causes fever, vomiting and continuous abdominal pain, which may not be localised to the right upper quadrant. Examination is therefore crucial in pinpointing the cause – right upper quadrant guarding (abdominal wall muscle resistance on examination) is the cardinal sign.

Action: Refer immediately to surgical admissions.

HIV medicine

Richard Hillman and Simon Barton

---

1 'Super bugs' are rare: if a patient has an unusually severe infection, think of immune suppression and HIV.

2 Mouth problems in a gay man warrant further investigation.

3 Needlestick injuries – hepatitis is more likely to be acquired than HIV.

4 A rash in an HIV-infected patient may be life-threatening.

5 Cough in an HIV-infected patient must be taken seriously.

6 Sudden change in vision in an HIV-infected patient could be blinding CMV retinitis.

NOTES

1 Atypical infections

Up to 40% of people with HIV in developed countries remain undiagnosed. They may present to primary care physicians with a range of fairly minor symptoms and signs associated with progressive immunosuppression. This can include genital warts that fail to respond to standard treatment or that recur very rapidly after therapy. Alternatively, patients may present with frequently recurrent and unusually severe herpes infection such as herpes simplex virus or varicella zoster virus. Multidermatomal zoster is particularly common. In women with recurrent candidiasis, the incidence of HIV may be up to four times higher.

An HIV antibody test must only be carried out with the individual's full consent and with adequate counselling both before and after the test has been performed.

Action: Consider immunosuppression in people with unusual or severe infections. Offer HIV testing widely.

2 Mouth problems in gay men

As a result of their sexual practices, gay men frequently have oral problems. Sore throat may be a result of acquiring an infection such as gonorrhoea (but this is commonly asymptomatic). Gingivitis and oral candidiasis may be a consequence of poor hygiene, or early indicators of immunosuppression from HIV. Oral hairy leukoplakia may present with a metal taste in the mouth and is one of the few pathognomonic features of HIV.

Action: Take a detailed sexual history and refer for sexually transmitted disease screening and possible HIV testing.

3 Needlestick injury

Patients who report needlestick injuries are frequently concerned about acquiring HIV. In most situations this is statistically unlikely, unless the needle is directly from a known

HIV-infected individual. A detailed personal risk activity history of the patient must be taken, together with specific information concerning the needlestick event. Knowledge of the local epidemiology of blood-borne viruses and their associated transmissibilities allows the approximate estimation of the likelihood of transmission. Typically, risk of transmission of hepatitis B (30%) and C (3%) are more common than HIV (0.3%). Passive and active immunisation against hepatitis B, and antiretroviral medications for HIV, may be effective if given soon after the event. Patients need to be aware of the possibility that they may be at risk of further onward transmission during the incubation period of the infections.

Action: Follow local protocols for risk determination, testing and prophylaxis. Advise the patient to practice safer sex until infection has been confidently excluded.

4 Hypersensitivity reaction

Rashes frequently occur in association with HIV. The commonest causes are medications and intercurrent infections. The immune dysregulation of HIV results in an increased frequency of drug allergies, including Stevens–Johnson syndrome. This may occur some considerable time after the drug has been introduced. Antiretroviral agents and other antimicrobials prescribed in HIV often have complex pharmacological interactions, which may be further complicated by non-prescribed therapies. Some drugs are more likely to cause rashes than others. Nevirapine often causes a rash. Abacavir can cause a life-threatening hypersensitivity reaction, of which rash may be a part.

Action: Take a good drug history. Refer immediately to the HIV clinic or dermatology.

5 Cough

Cough can be associated with typical and atypical infections in HIV. Where the immune system is well maintained, the cough should be managed in the standard manner. In the immunocompromised, *Pneumocystis carinii* pneumonia may present as a gradual reduction in exercise tolerance, unproductive cough and dyspnoea. Previously undiagnosed HIV infection often presents with this infection. As a result, HIV should be considered a cause of cough in those at risk. Pulmonary tuberculosis is more common in HIV, and may pose an infection control threat to staff and other patients.

Action: Refer urgently to the HIV clinic or chest clinic.

6 CMV retinitis

CMV infection is very common. In immunocompetent infections, CMV remains dormant after the initial infection (typically occurring in the late teen years). If the patient subsequently becomes immunocompromised as a result of HIV (or another cause), they are at risk of reactivation of their CMV. This can occur throughout the body, but the retina is the most vulnerable. The patient may present with floaters or a scotoma. Simple ophthalmoscope examination reveals the characteristic 'pizza pie' appearance with retinal haemorrhages and exudates. Retinal damage is irreversible once it has occurred, so rapid referral for specific antiviral treatment is essential to minimise permanent loss of sight.

Action: Refer immediately to ophthalmology.

Immunology

Gavin Spickett and Javier Carbone

1 Meningitis – more than once means there is an immune problem.

2 Recurrent, major infections could signify immunodeficiency.

3 Angio-oedema without urticaria in the young adult may be hereditary.

4 Angio-oedema without urticaria in an older adult may have associated systemic disease.

5 Sinus and nasal pain with red eyes could be Wegener's granulomatosis.

6 DVT with miscarriage or TIA – think of the antiphospholipid syndrome.

7 Not everyone with chronic fatigue has chronic fatigue syndrome.

8 In 'asthma' that is difficult to control, consider allergic aspergillosis.

9 Pregnancy in a woman with lupus or Sjögren's syndrome – risk of congenital heart block.

NOTES

1 Complement deficiency

Deficiency of complement component is associated with recurrent neisserial meningitis. Anyone with more than one episode of meningitis due to *N. meningitidis*, or a single episode with an unusual strain, needs urgent investigation. Non-immunological causes of recurrent meningitis also exist: the commonest is a connection between the CSF space and the exterior (usually via the sinuses). This can be difficult to identify.

Action: Refer urgently to immunology. For adults, give oral penicillin (or erythromycin if penicillin-sensitive) pending investigation.

2 Immunodeficiency

Recurrent or unusual infections are the hallmark of immuno-deficiency, both primary and secondary. Although, recurrent, minor, viral URTIs are not significant, proven, recurrent, bacterial or fungal infections should always be investigated. As a rule of thumb, two major infections in any 1 year (major = systemically unwell, requiring hospital admission and parenteral antibiotics) or one major and recurrent minor (all proven and requiring oral antibiotics) should be investigated. Also investigate any patient with deep-seated infection (e.g. osteo-myelitis, liver abscesses) or unusual organisms. Patients with unexplained bronchiectasis should also be investigated.

A baby under 1 year with infections and a blood count showing a lymphocyte count $< 2 \times 10^9/L$ may have severe combined immunodeficiency and must be discussed with a specialist paediatric immunologist.

Action: Refer urgently to immunology.

3 Hereditary angio-oedema (HAE)

Angio-oedema is characterised by acute attacks of subcutaneous oedema, commonly causing swelling of the perioral and periocular tissues. It usually presents in the context of urticaria, or skin weals. Angio-oedema occurring without urticaria, however, may be a symptom of HAE. Although genetic, this commonly does not present until adolescence. Swelling can be triggered by infection, stress and trauma, and can occur anywhere – bowel involvement can cause acute abdominal pain (surgery to be avoided). There may be a family history but new mutations are common. If urticaria is present, it is not HAE.

Action: Check complement C4 level (low/absent) and C1-esterase inhibitor (low/absent in Type I; normal or high in Type II) and refer to immunology.

4 Acquired angio-oedema

In an older person, HAE is less likely, and acquired angio-oedema more likely. The commonest cause is drug therapy, usually ACE inhibitors, statins and NSAIDs. It can develop any time after initiation of therapy. Rare associations are lymphoma, paraproteinaemia and connective tissue disease.

Action: Check drug therapy and stop likely culprits (may take several months for effect to disappear). If drugs are not suspected, examine for lymphadenopathy and splenomegaly, check serum immunoglobulins, serum and urinary electrophoresis and do an autoantibody screen for antinuclear antibodies (ANAs). Refer to immunology.

5 Wegener's granulomatosis

There are two types of Wegener's granulomatosis: one presenting with acute glomerulonephritis; and a more insidious form affecting predominantly upper and lower respiratory tract. Symptoms are usually persistent nasal discharge, epistaxis, sinus pain and red eyes. The combination of upper airway symptoms and ocular inflammation should raise suspicion. 95% of Wegener's patients will be positive for antineutrophil cytoplasmic antibodies (ANCAs), usually with antiproteinase-3 antibodies.

Action: Check ESR, CRP and ANCAs. Refer urgently to rheumatology or immunology. If eyes are involved, refer urgently to ophthalmology.

6 Antiphospholipid syndrome

A patient who has had miscarriages and venous thrombosis may have an underlying autoimmune disease, the antiphospholipid syndrome. The condition may also present as TIA or stroke in a young person. Treatment is lifelong warfarinisation. Aspirin has not been shown to be adequate. Untreated, there is risk of life-threatening complications (similar to disseminated intravascular coagulation), recurrent cerebral embolic events and progressive intellectual deterioration.

Action: Check for anticardiolipin antibodies and lupus anticoagulant (do both, as one alone may be negative). Check platelets (slightly reduced) and activated partial thromboplastin time (APTT) (prolonged). Refer to immunology.

7 Chronic fatigue

Presentations with chronic fatigue are common in all areas of medicine, but not all patients have chronic fatigue syndrome. Adrenal insufficiency regularly presents in this way (look for palmar and buccal pigmentation, and weight loss). In the overweight, consider sleep apnoea (check with family for snoring and apnoea). There is also an increased incidence of coeliac disease in patients presenting with fatigue.

Action: Check endomysial or tissue transglutaminase antibodies to exclude coeliac disease. If Addison's disease is suspected, refer to endocrinology. For sleep apnoea, arrange sleep studies.

8 Allergic bronchopulmonary aspergillosis (ABPA)

ABPA is a disease with the clinical features of asthma. Delay in diagnosis can lead to fibrosis and respiratory failure. ABPA should be suspected in asthmatics who are not well controlled on adequate bronchodilators, who are steroid-dependent, or who have recurrent pulmonary infiltrates on CXR. The total serum IgE concentration is markedly elevated, but is not specific. IgG and IgE serum antibodies to *Aspergillus fumigatus* are useful in diagnosis. High-resolution CT of the chest demonstrates multiple areas of bronchiectasis in most patients with ABPA. Prednisone remains the definitive treatment but need not be administered indefinitely. For patients with corticosteroid-dependent ABPA, the addition of itraconazole can help.

Action: Refer to respiratory medicine or immunology.

9 Congenital heart block (CHB)

CHB can occur with or without major structural cardiac abnormalities. If structural abnormalities are not present, the cause of CHB is thought to be autoimmune, showing a strong association with maternal antibodies to Ro (SS-A) and La (SS-B). Mothers with antibodies to Ro and La may have clinical or subclinical connective tissue disease (SLE, Sjögren's syndrome). CHB is most commonly diagnosed between 18 and 24 weeks of gestation, and may be first, second or third degree (complete). Mortality approaches approximately 20%, and most surviving children require pacemakers. In pregnant women with anti-Ro/La antibodies, serial echocardiographic analysis is therefore strongly recommended.

Action: Check anti-Ro/La antibodies in all SLE or Sjögren patients wishing to conceive.

Metabolic medicine

Jonathan Bodansky and Sadaf Farooqi

1 Abdominal or back pain in a newly diagnosed diabetic patient may signify pancreatic cancer.

2 A diabetic patient complaining of any foot infection, no matter how innocuous it looks, can lose their leg.

3 A type 1 diabetic patient with falling insulin requirements has an additional medical condition until proved otherwise.

4 Diarrhoea in a diabetic patient on metformin is due to this drug until proved otherwise.

5 A diabetic woman who becomes pregnant, or a pregnant woman who develops diabetes, is in danger of losing the baby.

6 Pruritus vulvae can be a presentation of diabetes in middle-aged women.

7 Deteriorating vision in a diabetic patient could herald sight-threatening retinopathy.

8 Vomiting and abdominal pain in a diabetic patient: consider life-threatening diabetic ketoacidosis.

9 Night sweats, seizures and morning headaches are symptoms of nocturnal hypoglycaemia.

10 Persistent nausea or vomiting with abdominal pain may be due to hypercalcaemia.

NOTES

1 Pancreatic cancer in a diabetic patient

Diabetes usually presents with a set of typical symptoms: thirst, polyuria, tiredness and weight loss. Pain is not a feature. In the occasional case, however, the presentation is with, or due to, cancer. Pancreatic cancer can present with diabetes, but usually also causes pain in the back, or upper abdominal pain radiating to the back, sometimes with disproportionate weight loss. CT of the pancreas is helpful in diagnosis.

Action: Refer urgently to medicine.

2 Diabetic foot infections

Foot infections in diabetic patients can go disastrously wrong. Probably the commonest reason why diabetic patients sue is for loss of a leg. Diabetic patients are prone to foot infections because they often have poor peripheral circulation and peripheral neuropathy. No matter how innocuous an infection appears, do not be fooled into thinking that it will respond to a single course of antibiotics. Proximal spread and gangrene may be rapid. When foot tissues go black, local amputation is usually ineffective, so below-knee amputation is often the outcome.

Action: Start oral antibiotics (e.g. flucloxacillin and ampicillin) and refer immediately to the diabetic clinic, preferably a diabetic foot clinic.

3 Falling insulin requirements

Repeated hypoglycaemia and falling insulin requirements in a type 1 diabetic patient usually means the patient has an additional medical condition. Consider coeliac disease, Addison's disease, thyroid disorder and hypopituitarism. These may all complicate type 1 diabetes. Malignancy may cause the same scenario, so this complaint should never be ignored.

Action: Check for coeliac disease, thyroid, adrenal and pituitary function, and look for clinical evidence of malignancy.

4 Metformin-related diarrhoea

Metformin is commonly used to treat diabetes. It has several modes of action, but works partly by causing carbohydrate malabsorption. This leads to its common side-effects of abdominal cramps or pain, increased flatus and diarrhoea. This diarrhoea can come on, not only when starting the drug, but even when patients have been on metformin for months or years, and had initially tolerated it. Considering this side-effect, needless colonoscopies or barium enemas can be prevented.

Action: Stop the metformin and wait 2 weeks. The diarrhoea is likely to resolve if it is due to the drug.

5 Diabetes and pregnancy

Pregnancy complicated by any type of diabetes is high risk. There is a danger of miscarriage, fetal death, macrosomia, complications of labour and fetal hypoglycaemia. Fetal malformation is more likely if the maternal blood glucose control is poor in the first trimester. Beware that a history of a large-for-dates baby or unexplained stillbirth may signify a tendency to gestational diabetes.

Action: Refer any diabetic woman who becomes pregnant to a combined, specialist clinic run by a diabetologist and an obstetrician within 1 week. Similarly, refer a pregnant lady who develops gestational diabetes. Refer a diabetic woman who is considering becoming pregnant to a combined clinic for prepregnancy counselling.

6 Pruritus vulvae

Type 2 diabetes causes a tendency to develop fungal infections in damp, occluded areas of the body, such as the vulva and vagina, under the prepuce and under the breasts. There is also a risk of soft tissue bacterial infections. These tendencies are related to an elevated blood glucose level. If a patient has pruritus vulvae, balanitis or submammary fungal infection, check for undiagnosed diabetes. The same applies for recurrent bacterial infections. Patients with type 2 diabetes probably have the condition for 8–10 years prior to diagnosis. Missed opportunities for diagnosis may allow the development of diabetic complications, which could have been prevented if diabetes had been considered.

Action: Check for diabetes (fasting glucose).

7 Diabetic retinopathy

Diabetes can damage the retina. The three main risk factors for this are the duration of diabetes, poor glucose control and high blood pressure. Retinopathy may regress with tight glucose and blood pressure control in its early stages, but sometimes requires laser therapy. However, it should be noted that early, treatable retinopathy does not usually cause symptoms. By the time retinopathy does cause visual loss, it is usually serious and may even be too late for useful treatment. As a result, a report of deteriorating vision should be taken seriously. Screening for retinopathy is mandatory to pick up changes at a treatable stage.

Action: Refer diabetic patients reporting falling vision urgently to ophthalmology. Ensure every diabetic patient you are responsible for receives annual screening for retinopathy.

8 Diabetic Ketoacidosis (DKA)

DKA usually presents with nausea, vomiting and cramping abdominal pain. It is one of the classical medical causes of the acute abdomen. At this early stage, it is usually confused with viral gastroenteritis. DKA can develop in any diabetic patient, whether on insulin or tablets, although more commonly in the insulin-dependent patient. It can be the first presenting complaint of an undiagnosed diabetic patient, and so should be considered even without a known history of diabetes, especially in younger patients. A patient with the textbook appearance of coma, dehydration and Kussmaul's respiration has severe DKA, which may be rapidly fatal.

Action: Check the blood glucose level and dipstick the urine for ketones. If blood glucose is raised, and urine is positive for ketones, refer immediately to the emergency department.

9 Nocturnal hypoglycaemia

Low blood glucose levels during the night are a common problem in patients treated with insulin. While they may be entirely asymptomatic, they can cause night sweats, morning headaches and seizures. Sweating during the day may also signify hypoglycaemia, but may alternatively be a feature of autonomic neuropathy or obesity. Apart from hypoglycaemia, epilepsy and space-occupying lesions should be considered in the differential diagnosis of seizures.

Action: Refer urgently to the diabetic clinic for adjustment of the insulin doses or regimen.

10 Hypercalcaemia

Hypercalcaemia is frequently associated with nausea, vomiting and abdominal pain, as well as constipation. Metabolic causes of these symptoms are often overlooked in favour of GI investigations, which are usually negative. All patients with these symptoms should have a serum calcium measurement. Common causes of hypercalcaemia include primary hyperparathyroidism and hypercalcaemia of malignancy. If serum calcium is elevated, a serum parathyroid hormone measurement will aid the differential diagnosis.

Action: Rehydrate with normal saline. Check parathyroid hormone, phosphate, ESR and serum protein electrophoresis (to rule out multiple myeloma) and do CXR (to look for bronchogenic carcinoma).

Neurology

Andrew Larner, Graham Niepel and Cris Constantinescu

1 Transient, bilateral loss of vision suggests raised intracranial pressure.

2 All oculomotor (third nerve) palsies are urgent, whether the pupil is involved or not.

3 Worsening neurological symptoms in the evening suggests myasthenia gravis.

4 Episodic loss of consciousness without provoking factors may be due to epilepsy.

5 Numb chin – think of metastatic carcinoma.

6 Progressive headache with neck stiffness, fever, vomiting, with or without rash, is bacterial meningitis until proved otherwise.

7 Do not forget viral encephalitis in the elderly with pyrexia and altered level of consciousness.

8 Sensory disturbance on neck flexion suggests an inflammatory lesion of the cervical spinal cord.

9 Thunderclap headache or focal neurology during pregnancy or post partum may mean cerebral venous sinus thrombosis.

10 Progressive ascending paralysis may be caused by Guillain–Barré syndrome.

NOTES

1 Raised intracranial pressure (ICP)

Transient bilateral loss of vision ('greying out') lasting a few seconds, particularly if associated with an activity known to raise ICP (coughing, sneezing, bending down or straining at stool), suggests critical compromise of optic nerve head perfusion. Other symptoms of raised ICP may be present, such as early morning or recumbent headache, associated with nausea and vomiting. Papilloedema on fundoscopy confirms the clinical diagnosis. Management involves neuroimaging to exclude a space-occupying lesion and prompt treatment to reduce ICP and prevent permanent visual loss.

Action: Refer immediately to neurology.

2 Oculomotor (third nerve) palsy

Oculomotor (third nerve) palsy presents with diplopia, often with eye pain. Examination may show ptosis, ophthalmoplegia in all directions other than lateral gaze, with or without pupil enlargement. The proposed distinction of 'surgical' causes (e.g. posterior communicating artery aneurysm) from 'medical' causes (e.g. infarction associated with diabetes or hypertension) on the basis of pupil involvement (surgical) or sparing (medical) should not be relied upon. Neuroimaging is required.

Action: Refer immediately to neurology.

3 Myasthenia gravis (MG)

Complaints of weakness or fatigue may reflect either a subjective sensation of tiredness or objective weakness. The variable weakness of MG is suggested by worsening of symptoms towards the end of the day and improvement with rest (the 'sleep test' has been suggested for the diagnosis of MG). Myasthenic weakness is fatigable, i.e. objectively worsened by repeated muscle contraction. Tests for fatigability include prolonged upgaze leading to ptosis and diplopia, counting out loud leading to hypophonia, or repeated proximal limb movements ('wing beats') leading to reduced power. Respiratory muscle weakness is best assessed by spirometry, but is suggested clinically by shortness of breath on lying down and inability to complete sentences.

Action: Refer urgently to neurology, immediately if there is evidence of respiratory involvement.

4 Epilepsy

Episodic loss of consciousness is diagnostically challenging. The main differential is between epilepsy and syncope. Diagnosis is essentially clinical, based on the description of attacks – electroencephalogram (EEG) cannot confirm or refute a diagnosis of epilepsy. Clinical history may rely on eyewitness reports. Premonitory symptoms of light-headedness, 'distancing' of vision or hearing, sweating and pallor are more suggestive of syncope. This condition may be associated with myoclonic jerking movements, which may be misinterpreted as a 'convulsion' or 'fit', although they differ from the tonic-clonic movements typical of a generalised epileptic seizure. Incontinence may occur in either epileptic seizure or syncope. Prolonged (> 20 min) post-event confusion is more suggestive of an epileptic seizure.

Action: Refer to neurology if epilepsy is suspected – some centres have dedicated 'first fit' clinics. Give advice on driving, following DVLA guidelines.

5 Numb chin

Facial numbness or paraesthesiae confined to the chin indicates a trigeminal neuropathy (mental nerve branch) secondary to metastatic carcinoma until proved otherwise.

Action: Enquire about any history of dental surgery or trauma and assess for sites of a possible primary. Refer urgently to neurology or medicine.

6 Bacterial meningitis

Fever, malaise, headache, neck stiffness, irritability and confusion developing over hours to a day or two are the typical features of bacterial meningitis. Always look for a petechial/purpuric, non-blanching rash, suggesting a diagnosis of meningococcal septicaemia. In the very young, very old, or immunosuppressed patients, typical features such as meningism may be lacking – an increased index of clinical suspicion is therefore required in these groups. Prior antibiotic use may also mask the severity of the illness.

Action: Refer immediately. If meningococcal meningitis is suspected, give IV/IM benzylpenicillin before transfer to hospital.

7 Viral encephalitis

Elderly patients frequently present with confusion or drowsiness with pyrexia. Common causes include UTI and LRTI. However, it is important not to forget that encephalitis may present in the same way. More suspicious features include headache, seizures, dysphasia or any focal neurological deficit. Viral encephalitis is seen more in children and young adults, but in these age groups there is a much higher index of suspicion. In fact, encephalitis can occur at any age. Management involves septic screen and consideration of neuroimaging followed by lumbar puncture.

Action: Perform a detailed history and examination looking for sources of infection. Dipstick the urine. Refer immediately to medicine.

8 Lhermitte's sign

Lhermitte's sign refers to a brief sensory disturbance that passes down the back, sometimes involving the limbs, upon neck flexion. Typical sensations include an electric shock–like sensation and paraesthesiae. It is most commonly found in multiple sclerosis and is secondary to a demyelinating lesion within the cervical spinal cord. Similar symptoms that occur upon neck extension are thought, most commonly, to be secondary to a cervical myelopathy. Typical neuropathic pain treatments, such as anticonvulsants or tricyclic antidepressants, may be of benefit.

Action: Refer to neurology.

9 Cerebral venous sinus thrombosis

Some neurological conditions are more common during pregnancy, such as Bell's palsy or carpal tunnel syndrome. Cerebral venous sinus thrombosis is a rare but potentially life-threatening condition that makes up a higher proportion of 'strokes' in pregnancy or the immediate post-partum period. Headache is commonly reported and may be an acute thunderclap headache similar to subarachnoid haemorrhage. Other common presenting complaints include disorders of consciousness and seizures. Focal neurological signs in pregnancy or post partum, especially in conjunction with a headache, should raise suspicions.

Action: Refer immediately to neurology.

10 Guillain-Barré syndrome (GBS)

The early diagnosis of GBS may be difficult. It can present with insidious onset of distal paraesthesiae and variable weakness, sometimes with abdominal pain, evolving over a period of days. There may be a history of preceding infection, especially gastrointestinal. Limb weakness is typically symmetrical, in a 'pyramidal' distribution, often ascending from lower to upper limbs, and there may also be facial weakness. Tendon reflexes are usually absent. Diaphragm involvement may lead to life-threatening respiratory compromise. Autonomic features may occur, such as cardiac arrhythmia and urinary retention.

Action: Refer immediately to neurology.

Neurosurgery

Stana Bojanic, Richard Kerr, Guy Wynne-Jones and Jonathan Wasserberg

1 Sudden onset of headache – think of subarachnoid haemorrhage.

2 Reduced level of consciousness after head injury may be due to extradural haematoma.

3 An elderly patient with confusion, hemiparesis or deteriorating consciousness level after a fall – exclude chronic subdural haematoma.

4 Continuing complaints of headache, worse in the morning, may indicate raised intracranial pressure.

5 New onset of seizures in an adult means a brain tumour until proved otherwise.

6 Low back pain with sphincter disturbance is cauda equina syndrome until proved otherwise.

7 Sudden onset of headache, visual deterioration and reduced mental state may be pituitary apoplexy.

8 Headache with eye movement abnormality requires a scan.

9 Clear fluid leaking from the nose or ear after trauma may be CSF.

10 A patient with difficulty walking – check for a sensory level.

NOTES

1 Subarachnoid haemorrhage (SAH)

Most SAHs present with sudden onset of severe headache (like being hit with a 'hammer') unlike anything the patient has ever experienced. There may be transient loss of consciousness followed by recovery. Nausea, vomiting, neck stiffness and photophobia may occur. In many cases, the patient is able to carry on with what they were doing before, but may then feel increasingly unwell. In all cases of sudden onset of headache, think of SAH first, irrespective of the speed of recovery. CT is used for diagnosis but may initially be normal in a small percentage of cases – lumbar puncture is required for these.

Action: Resuscitate if necessary. Refer immediately to neurosurgery.

2 Extradural haematoma (EDH)

The classical presentation of EDH is brief loss of consciousness after head injury, followed by a lucid interval and then further deterioration. The presence of scalp laceration, boggy swelling or skull fracture is associated with increased risk of deterioration. There may be hemiparesis (often ipsilateral to the side of the EDH, a false localising sign) or a dilated pupil. EDH normally originates from a torn middle meningeal artery, with blood clot developing between the bone and the dura. Urgent clot evacuation is required.

Action: Intubate and ventilate if necessary. Arrange emergency CT scan, and refer immediately to neurosurgery.

3 Chronic subdural haematoma

Chronic subdural haematoma is common in elderly patients, due to a combination of cerebral atrophy and falls. It is also commonly not diagnosed for several weeks after onset of symptoms. Typically, the patient develops increasing confusion, possibly weakness of an arm or leg, without associated headache. As the condition progresses over weeks, or months, the patient's consciousness level may start to fluctuate. There is often a history of previous trauma, which may be mild and not fully appreciated. CT shows up the haematoma well.

Action: Arrange urgent CT and refer urgently to neurosurgery. Check clotting and try to stop anticoagulants or aspirin.

4 Raised intracranial pressure (ICP)

Increasingly severe headaches in a previously healthy patient should prompt further investigation for an intracranial lesion. Worrying associated features are papilloedema and vomiting, which complete the triad of raised ICP. Urinary incontinence can also occur.

Action: Arrange urgent neuroimaging and refer urgently to neurosurgery.

5 New seizures

New onset of seizures in an adult suggests a space-occupying lesion in the brain, until proved otherwise. Seizures are the most common form of presentation of a low-grade glioma or arteriovenous malformation in a young adult. Other causes are head injury, infection, congenital abnormalities or acute systemic metabolic disturbance.

Action: Arrange urgent neuroimaging and refer urgently to neurology or neurosurgery.

6 Cauda equina syndrome

In a patient with low back pain radiating to both legs, it is essential to ensure that sphincter function is normal. Patients can be unaware that they have lost urinary sphincter function, or have lost sensation and tone in the anal sphincter. Specifically ask if the patient has passed urine. Examination is mandatory to ensure that perineal and perianal sensation, as well as anal tone, are normal. Failure to detect loss of sphincter function early on can result in permanent incontinence. Causes of cauda equina syndrome include intervertebral disc prolapse, compression by tumour, or trauma.

Action: Refer immediately to neurosurgery or orthopaedics.

7 Pituitary apoplexy

Pituitary apoplexy is infarction or haemorrhage in a pituitary tumour and can cause life-threatening hypopituitarism. It usually presents with headache, visual loss, ophthalmoplegia and reduced mental state. However, associated cavernous sinus compression can cause trigeminal nerve symptoms or proptosis. Neuroimaging shows a haemorrhagic mass in the sella turcica and/or suprasellar region. Pituitary function is always compromised, necessitating rapid administration of corticosteroids and endocrine evaluation.

Action: Refer immediately to neurosurgery with endocrinology input.

8 Midbrain mass lesion

Any patient with new headache and new eye movement abnormality needs neuroimaging. Increasingly severe headache and failure of upgaze may point to insidious onset of hydrocephalus. Patients with a pineal tumour, for instance, often present with 6–8 weeks of headache, followed by double vision. Eye movement examination may reveal loss of upgaze and failure of convergence (Parinaud's syndrome).

Action: Check for papilloedema and arrange urgent MRI. Refer urgently to neurology or neurosurgery.

9 CSF leak

Leak of CSF can follow trauma or surgery. Spontaneous leak is rare. Following trauma, CSF leak is associated with meningitis in up to 10% of cases. *Streptococcus pneumoniae* is the most common pathogen. The first step is to establish that the leaking fluid is actually CSF. The fluid is clear and may taste salty. If possible collect fluid for testing. Glucose strips are very sensitive and may be positive even with excess mucus. The most sensitive test for CSF is the β2-transferrin test.

Action: If possible, collect fluid for testing. Refer immediately to neurosurgery.

10 Spinal cord compression

Spinal cord compression is commonly missed in its early stages and is not usually diagnosed until the patient is unable to walk. The patient who is complaining of difficulty walking and standing should be carefully examined to rule out spinal cord compression. In particular, look for a sensory level on the trunk.

Action: Arrange urgent MRI and refer urgently to neurosurgery.

Obstetrics

Chandrima Biswas, Christina Cotzias and Philip Steer

In a pregnant woman:

1 Headache, flashing lights and epigastric pain means pre-eclampsia until proved otherwise.

2 Vaginal bleeding must always be investigated.

3 Haemoptysis, shortness of breath or chest pain suggest pulmonary embolism.

4 Calf pain or swelling – always investigate for DVT.

5 Watery vaginal discharge may signal preterm prelabour rupture of the membranes.

6 Severe itching, especially of the palms and soles, may be due to obstetric cholestasis.

7 Do not miss preterm labour.

8 When a woman says that her baby is not moving as usual, take her seriously.

9 Continuous, worsening lower abdominal pain may indicate placental abruption.

10 Multiple changing, trivial complaints, or missed appointments, may flag up psychological or social problems, including domestic violence.

NOTES

1 Pre-eclampsia

If a pregnant woman complains of headache, visual disturbance ('flashing lights') and epigastric pain, pre-eclampsia must be excluded. Vomiting and oedema of the hands and face may also occur. Pre-eclampsia can cause maternal death, and is a risk factor for many major obstetric emergencies. It is classically described as hypertension and proteinuria of new onset in the second half of pregnancy. The only cure is delivery.

Action: Check BP carefully. Dipstick the urine for protein. If BP ≥ 140/90, or if there is more than a trace of proteinuria, arrange immediate admission (by ambulance) to a maternity unit.

2 Placenta praevia

Any vaginal bleeding in the second half of pregnancy is serious. Causes include placenta praevia, placental abruption, preterm labour or even an undiagnosed cervical cancer. Placenta praevia is where the placenta is implanted close to, or covering, the cervix, classically causing painless vaginal bleeding. Often small, self-resolving warning bleeds precede a heavier bleed. These women are at risk of massive obstetric haemorrhage, both antenatally and post partum.

Action: Do *not* perform a digital vaginal examination. In severe haemorrhage, insert at least two wide-bore peripheral IV lines and start rescuscitation. Send off FBC and cross-match. Call obstetric service immediately. For minor bleeds, it is essential to establish more accurately the amount and source of bleeding, so a speculum (not digital) examination must be carried out by an appropriately qualified doctor. Check fetal well-being by cardiotocography.

3 Pulmonary embolism (PE)

In patients with haemoptysis, acute shortness of breath, chest pain or severe cough, PE should always be at the top of the list.

Thromboembolism is a leading direct cause of maternal death in the UK. The risk remains high even in the first 6 postnatal weeks. Investigations for PE (CXR, VQ scans or spiral CT scan) are not contraindicated in pregnancy.

Action: Refer immediately for assessment and treatment. If there is clinical suspicion, commence treatment with sub-cutaneous low–molecular weight heparin or IV unfractionated heparin until the diagnosis is excluded by objective testing.

4 DVT

Although leg oedema, unilateral or bilateral, is a common feature of pregnancy, DVT must always be considered. Left-sided DVT is nine times more common than right-sided DVT. Classical signs of leg swelling, erythema, pain and tenderness of the calf are unreliable, so a high index of suspicion is necessary. If a positive diagnosis is made, women should wear thromboembolic deterrent (TED) stockings for 2 years to minimise the risk of post-thrombotic syndrome.

Action: Refer immediately to obstetrics or via local DVT protocols.

5 Preterm prelabour rupture of the membranes (PPROM)

Many women complain of increased vaginal loss ('feeling damp') in pregnancy. This could be physiological or due to urinary incontinence. However, PPROM must not be missed. The concerns are premature delivery (many women will go into labour spontaneously within 48 h) and the risk, to fetus and mother, of ascending infection. Women can develop overwhelming sepsis insidiously and quickly, and fever or tachycardia in these patients must be taken seriously.

Action: Do a sterile speculum examination with the mother in a recumbent position, to check for the presence of a pool of liquor. If this is observed, refer immediately to obstetrics.

6 Obstetric cholestasis

Itching in pregnancy is common and usually benign. Obstetric cholestasis must always be considered, however, as it can lead to a sudden intrauterine death (usually after 37 weeks of gestation), as well as preterm labour and postpartum haemorrhage. The characteristic feature is severe itching on the limbs, trunk, palms and soles of the feet, often so severe that it disrupts sleep. Although there is no associated rash, scratch marks are often evident. LFTs are abnormal and serum total bile acid (BA) concentrations are increased. There may be vitamin K deficiency because of malabsorption of fat-soluble vitamins.

Action: Check LFTs and serum BA. Refer urgently to obstetrics.

7 Preterm labour

The diagnosis of labour is important at term, but is vital pre-term, as preterm delivery is responsible for 80% of neonatal deaths. Abdominal pain coming for 30 s, every 2–10 min, and getting worse, is labour, until proved otherwise. In addition, constant backache, pelvic heaviness or increased vaginal discharge, which is mucous or bloody, should also ring alarm bells. Always think: has pre-term labour started, and if so, why? The only way to diagnose labour with certainty is to observe progressive dilatation of the cervix. Thus, a vaginal examination should always be performed if preterm labour is suspected.

Action: Do a vaginal examination. Refer immediately to a maternity unit if the cervix is not long and closed.

8 Intrauterine death

Although there is no good evidence for the use of 'kick charts', when a mother spontaneously reports reduced or absent fetal movement, take her seriously. It may indicate fetal hypoxia or death. The absolute priority is to detect fetal heart activity. If not detected, it is wise to obtain an experienced second opinion, because erroneously telling a woman her baby has died, when in fact it is still alive, is traumatic both for both parents and doctor. Furthermore, parents may need the second opinion to accept the news.

Action: Check for fetal heart activity using a portable Doppler. (Do not accept arterial pulsations alone, as this may be maternal. Always search for the characteristic, multiple signals from the heart.) Always monitor for several minutes, because occasionally a severe bradycardia can give the impression of cardiac asystole. Refer immediately to obstetrics if heart activity is not detected.

9 Placental abruption

Severe abruption is partial or complete separation of the placenta from the uterus and is a true obstetric emergency. It usually presents with pain and vaginal bleeding, but the bleeding can be concealed. The pain is variable, and if severe, may be associated with sweating, agitation and even vomiting. If the placenta is posterior, backache may be the presenting complaint. Women can become very unwell, very quickly, with cardiovascular compromise or coagulopathy. In an extensive abruption there may be fetal hypoxia or even death.

Action: Insert two wide-bore peripheral lines and commence resuscitation. Refer immediately to obstetrics.

10 Domestic violence

Women who repeatedly attend antenatal clinics, GP surgeries or emergency departments with medically trivial complaints may have serious psychological problems or social difficulties, or may be victims of domestic violence. Abuse against women unfortunately often escalates in pregnancy. It can cause depression, alcohol and drug abuse, miscarriage, stillbirth, severe maternal morbidity and even maternal death either by suicide or murder. Alarm bells should also ring when a woman misses appointments, self-discharges or is reluctant to speak in front of her partner. Domestic violence is more likely to be detected by direct and repeated questioning by health professionals.

Action: Ask about relationships, especially with partners. Make available printed information about how to get help – women's toilets are a good place to supply it discreetly. Contact the maternity unit and speak to the designated member of staff responsible for the care of women suffering from domestic violence.

Oncology

Robin Jones and Ian Smith

1 Do not ignore a fever or flulike symptoms in a patient on chemotherapy.

2 Gradual increase in abdominal girth in a middle-aged woman may be due to ovarian cancer.

3 Dyspnoea in a cancer patient could mean pulmonary emboli.

4 Painless lymphadenopathy with systemic symptoms could be due to lymphoma or metastases.

5 A plethoric face and facial swelling could be due to superior vena cava obstruction.

6 Back pain in a young man could be due to testicular cancer.

7 Hoarse voice with difficulty breathing is suspicious for a mediastinal tumour.

8 Diplopia can be a presenting feature of orbital or central nervous system metastases.

9 Morning headaches could indicate cerebral metastases.

10 Unexplained weight loss of more than 10% in a middle-aged person could be a sign of malignancy.

NOTES

1 Neutropenic sepsis

Neutropenic sepsis occurs due to the myelosuppressive effect of cytotoxic chemotherapy. Any patient undergoing chemotherapy who presents with a fever, together with signs and symptoms of infection, should be considered neutropenic. The nadir typically occurs 7–10 days following cytotoxic therapy, although it can occur earlier or later. This is a life-threatening condition and requires prompt action. Management includes IV antibiotics.

Action: Refer immediately to oncology.

2 Ovarian cancer

Women with ovarian cancer often present late due to the anatomical location of the ovaries. A middle-aged female with unexplained increase in abdominal girth may have ascites, which could be due to ovarian cancer.

Action: A full examination should be performed with particular attention paid to the abdominal system. Refer urgently.

3 Pulmonary emboli

Due to changes in the coagulation system and possibly occasional vessel stasis, cancer patients have a predisposition to develop DVT and pulmonary emboli. Any oncology patient presenting with progressive or acute shortness of breath and pleuritic chest pain should be suspected as having a pulmonary embolus.

Action: Refer immediately to medical admissions.

4 Lymphoma

There are many causes of lymphadenopathy, but in conjunction with systemic features such as night sweats, fevers, weight loss, pruritus and lethargy, lymphoma must be considered.

Action: Perform a full examination looking for lymphadenopathy elsewhere and hepatosplenomegaly. Refer urgently to medicine.

5 Superior vena cava obstruction

Compression of the superior vena cava occurs most commonly in lung cancer and lymphoma, as well as breast and kidney cancer. Patients complain of facial swelling, a sensation of fullness in the head and shortness of breath.

Action: Refer immediately for CXR and further investigation by a respiratory team.

6 Testicular cancer

Although rare, testicular cancer is still the commonest solid tumour in men aged between 15 and 34 years. The primary tumour usually presents as a painless, progressively enlarging lump in the scrotum. The first presentation, however, can be back pain due to retroperitoneal lymphadenopathy from metastatic disease. Testicular tumours are particularly sensitive to chemotherapy and are usually curable.

Action: Refer urgently to urology.

7 Mediastinal tumours

Recent onset of hoarseness can be due to palsy of the recurrent laryngeal nerve. If a new onset of hoarse voice is accompanied by other respiratory symptoms (dyspnoea, chest tightness or pain), the cause could be a mediastinal tumour.

Action: Perform a full examination with particular attention to the respiratory system. Refer urgently to the chest clinic.

8 Orbital and central nervous system metastases

Most diplopia is not due to tumours. However, in a patient with a history of cancer who complains of double vision, metastasis to the orbit or central nervous system should be considered. Investigation with CT or MRI of the brain will clarify the location of the lesion.

Action: Perform a full neurological examination. Refer urgently to oncology.

9 Raised intracranial pressure (ICP)

Early morning headaches may be the presenting symptom of cerebral metastases resulting in raised ICP. Other features could be vomiting (with no nausea), altered consciousness, convulsions and occasionally protracted nausea with no vomiting.

Action: Check pulse (low), BP (high) and examine for focal neurological signs, especially papilloedema. Refer immediately to neurology or oncology.

10 Weight loss

Unexplained weight loss in a middle-aged person could be a sign of malignancy. Loss of more than 10% of the original weight is suspicious. Other symptoms and signs that could give an indication of the underlying cause should be sought. These could include change in bowel habit, rectal bleeding, pain, any palpable masses and shortness of breath or cough.

Action: Perform a full clinical evaluation, including a rectal examination. Refer urgently to the appropriate team.

Ophthalmology

Nadeem Ali, Philip Griffiths and Scott Fraser

1 Do not forget giant cell arteritis in any patient over 50 with sudden visual loss, even without pain.

2 Painful, red eye with vomiting – think of acute glaucoma.

3 Falling vision with pain after cataract surgery is intraocular infection until proved otherwise.

4 An unwell child with tender, puffy lids may develop intracranial infection.

5 Flashes and floaters are potential symptoms of retinal detachment.

6 Sudden onset of double vision may herald life-threatening neurology.

7 Eye trauma that is high-velocity or from a sharp object – rule out penetrating injury.

8 Sticky eyes in a neonate could be sight-threatening.

9 A white pupil in a child is a life-threatening tumour until proved otherwise.

10 Thyroid eye disease can cause blindness.

NOTES

1 Giant cell arteritis (GCA)

Always think of GCA (= superficial temporal arteritis) in patients over 50 who complain of visual loss without eye pain. Untreated, the central retinal arteries can occlude and the patient can be blind in both eyes within a day. Other symptoms to ask about include headache, temple pain, scalp tenderness (pain on brushing hair), jaw claudication (pain on chewing), muscle stiffness, weight loss and fever. Occasionally, none of these symptoms are present (occult GCA). CRP is more sensitive a test than ESR. Superficial temporal artery biopsy can confirm the diagnosis and is not affected by prior steroid treatment.

Action: Check confrontation fields, feel the temporal arteries (hard, tender or pulseless). Do ESR, CRP and FBC. Refer immediately to ophthalmology (to rheumatology if GCA without visual symptoms). Start high-dose per oral prednisolone (or IV hydrocortisone) if the picture fits.

2 Acute closed-angle glaucoma (ACAG)

ACAG can blind if left untreated. It classically presents with a unilateral painful red eye, with malaise and nausea. Sufferers are usually 'long-sighted' – they wear glasses that magnify their eyes. Occasionally, the presenting symptom can be vomiting with abdominal pain or headache. ACAG can be misdiagnosed, therefore, as an acute abdomen or as an intracranial event. Some patients report a few weeks or months of episodes of pain and misting of the vision in the evenings, with haloes or rainbows around lights. These represent intermittent, subacute attacks. The crucial sign is a fixed, mid-dilated pupil. If the pupil constricts normally to light, ACAG is practically excluded.

Action: Refer immediately to ophthalmology. Give IV acetazolamide if there is any delay in transfer. For history of intermittent attacks only, refer urgently.

3 Postsurgical endophthalmitis

Falling vision following intraocular surgery sets an ophthalmologist's pulse racing. Endophthalmitis is a microbial intraocular infection that can permanently destroy the vision. It is a rare complication of any intraocular procedure, most commonly cataract surgery. Falling vision and increasing pain are typical. Other suspicious signs are floaters, increasing photophobia and discharge.

Action: Refer immediately to ophthalmology.

4 Orbital cellulitis

If a child (or even adult) with tender, puffy eyelids is unwell, consider orbital cellulitis. The risk is intracranial spread of infection causing cavernous sinus thrombosis and meningitis. Headache, pyrexia, reduced vision, proptosis and limited, painful eye movements are suggestive features. The absence of systemic symptoms makes preseptal cellulitis (where the infection is confined to the superficial tissues) more likely.

Action: Check the temperature. Refer immediately to ophthalmology, urgently in the absence of systemic features.

5 Retinal detachment

Floaters are opacities in the vitreous cavity. They shift on movements of the eyes and get in the way of the vision. Patients describe them as dots, circles, cobwebs, hairs. They are often accompanied by flashing lights, like white sparkles, in the periphery of the visual field. Flashes and floaters are symptoms of an almost universal, and mostly benign, condition (posterior vitreous detachment), but also of a sight-threatening condition – retinal detachment. History alone cannot distinguish between the two. If the patient also reports a 'shadow' coming across their vision over hours or days (not minutes), retinal detachment should be assumed.

Action: Refer all new onset of flashes and floaters urgently to ophthalmology; immediately if accompanied by field loss or reduced vision.

6 Diplopia

Sudden onset of double vision may herald life-threatening neurology. The most serious cause is a painful third nerve (oculomotor) palsy, which may be caused by an aneurysm of the posterior communicating artery. The signs are limited elevation, depression and adduction, with ptosis. The axiom that an unaffected pupil excludes a compressive cause should not be relied upon.

A sixth nerve palsy causes limitation of abduction. It may be a false localising sign in raised intracranial pressure.

Palsy of the fourth cranial nerve is harder to diagnose, but it rarely indicates life-threatening disease. It may cause vertical diplopia, which increases on looking to one side, and reduces on looking to the other side.

Action: For third nerve palsies with pain and pupil involvement, refer immediately to neurosurgery. In other cases, refer immediately to ophthalmology or neurology.

7 Penetrating eye injury

Anyone who gives a history of ocular trauma followed by reduced vision needs full ophthalmic assessment. Sudden onset of 'floaters' is also worrying. The history of the event is crucial – certain scenarios, however trivial they may sound, should ring alarm bells. High-velocity impacts such as metal striking metal (hammer on chisel) have a high incidence of penetrating fragments. Sharp objects are worrying – broken glass, metal, wood, plastic. Have a lower threshold of suspicion in children where history may not be accurate. The eye may appear grossly normal – refer on the basis of history alone.

Action: Refer immediately to ophthalmology. Put a shield or pad over the eye – do not let it touch the eyeball.

8 Ophthalmia neonatorum

Ophthalmia neonatorum is conjunctivitis within the first month of life. The commonest causes are staphylococcal and streptococcal infections, which are either self-limiting or respond quickly to topical antibiotics. *Chlamydia* is increasingly common and can easily be overlooked. Gonococcus is the most serious cause, as it progress very rapidly and can lead to corneal perforation – it is therefore sight-threatening. Rarely, fulminant systemic infection develops. Both *chlamydia* and gonococcus are contracted from the mother during delivery. Purulent discharge within the first week of life is gonococcal until proved otherwise. Chlamydial conjunctivitis tends to present in the second week.

Action: Refer immediately to ophthalmology or paediatrics. Parents may need genitourinary investigations. Ophthalmia neonatorum is a notifiable disease.

9 Leukocoria

A white pupil (leukocoria) is often first noticed by parents looking at photographs of their children in which a normal 'red eye' is missing. There are many causes of leukocoria, the most serious of which is retinoblastoma, a life-threatening tumour.

Action: Confirm the loss of the normal, red pupil reflex with a direct ophthalmoscope from a distance. Refer urgently to ophthalmology.

10 Thyroid eye disease

Thyroid eye disease can occur in any thyroid state (hypo-, eu-, or hyper-) and the classical appearance is familiar to most doctors. A report of falling vision is worrying. The condition can cause sight loss either through corneal exposure and ulceration, or through optic nerve compression at the orbital apex. The former is more likely with obviously proptotic eyes, but the latter without obvious proptosis, so the first glance should not reassure.

Action: Check visual acuity and colour vision. Refer immediately to ophthalmology.

Oral and maxillofacial surgery

John Langdon and Robert Ord

1 Difficulty in opening the mouth – think of life-threatening infection.

2 Progressive difficulty swallowing and breathing – think of life-threatening infection.

3 Tongue pain that radiates to the ear is likely to be due to an invading cancer.

4 A mouth ulcer that lasts for more than 2 weeks is cancer until proved otherwise.

5 Red or white patches in the mouth could be malignant – even if not ulcerated.

6 A patient under 40 years with sharp, unilateral facial pain, or persistent facial paraesthesia, could have sinister trigeminal nerve pathology.

7 Swollen, bleeding gums in an anaemic patient could mean leukaemia.

8 Progressive facial palsy over a period of weeks is often malignant in origin.

9 Unilateral numb lip needs exclusion of malignancy.

10 Non-healing ulceration of the roof of the mouth could be lethal.

NOTES

1 Trismus

Trismus is difficulty in opening the jaws due to reflex muscle spasm and is a relatively common symptom. However, it is an alarm bell for life-threatening infections or tumours. Infection in the submasseteric space or in the pterygoid space will result in profound trismus often in the absence of significant pain or external swelling. The origin of the infection may be a partially erupted wisdom tooth or a simple dental abscess. The infection can cause airway compromise and may track into the mediastinum or up to the skull base. Intravenous antibiotics and emergency drainage under general anaesthesia are required. Painless trismus can also be caused by malignant tumours of the oropharynx, tonsil or maxillary sinus invading the masticatory muscles.

Action: Refer immediately to maxillofacial surgery.

2 Submandibular and sublingual infection

Ludwig's angina is a life-threatening spreading cellulitis involving the sublingual and submandibular spaces on both sides. The risk is of the rapid spread of infection and accompanying oedema into adjacent tissue spaces leading to respiratory obstruction and difficulty swallowing. In addition, the oedema can elevate the tongue, which impacts on the palate causing additional difficulty breathing. Spread of the infection posteriorly results in profound trismus. Airway management and surgical decompression are required. Intravenous antibiotics are needed too, but will not be successful without drainage.

Action: Refer immediately to maxillofacial surgery. Avoid tracheostomy if possible as this opens up further tissue spaces leading to the mediastinum.

3 Squamous cell carcinoma

Although otalgia is a common symptom from aural or temporomandibular joint disorders, it can be due to radiated pain from posterior tongue or oropharyngeal lesions. As a result, in patients complaining of ear pain with no obvious cause, the mouth and oropharynx should be examined. The lesions are usually deeply infiltrating squamous cell carcinomas involving the lingual nerve. If confirmed, radical surgery including neck dissection and post-operative radiotherapy may be needed.

Action: Refer urgently to maxillofacial surgery as a 'suspected cancer'.

4 Oral cancer

The tongue and floor of mouth are the two most common sites for oral cancer. Any patient who complains of a lesion, lump or ulcer at these sites present for more than 2 weeks should be suspected of having oral cancer. As opposed to common aphthous ulcers, which normally clear in about ten days, malignant lesions are solitary, large and can be initially painless. Although risk factors for oral cancer include tobacco and alcohol, non-smokers and patients under 40 years may also be affected. Biopsy is necessary.

Action: Refer urgently to maxillofacial surgery as a 'suspected cancer'.

5 Erythroplakia and leukoplakia

Erythroplakia (red patch) and leukoplakia (white patch) on the oral mucosa are premalignant lesions. The incidence of malignant change in an erythroplakia approaches 100%, whereas in a leukoplakia it is less than 10%. Suspicion should be heightened if the patient abuses tobacco or alcohol, but non-smokers who have never drunk alcohol can also be affected. All such lesions require definitive diagnosis by biopsy and long-term follow-up to detect malignant change at an early stage.

Action: Refer urgently to maxillofacial surgery.

6 Trigeminal nerve lesions

Severe, unilateral facial pain, which is sharp and lasts a few seconds, is the classic symptom of trigeminal neuralgia. Pain can be severe enough to make the patient suicidal. Most cases occur in elderly patients and are idiopathic. In a patient under 40 years an underlying condition, such as multiple sclerosis or tumour, should be suspected. Alternatively, persistent paraesthesia in the face or mouth can also herald serious trigeminal nerve pathology, such as a neural sheath tumour.

Action: Refer urgently to neurology or maxillofacial surgery.

7 Leukaemia

Swollen, bleeding gums are a very common manifestation of periodontal disease and occur in a sizeable proportion of the population. However, in a young patient who is unwell, looks anaemic and has new onset of swollen gums the physician should rule out an underlying leukemia. The gingiva can become stuffed with blast cells in this condition.

Action: Check FBC.

8 Facial palsy

Bell's palsy is of relatively rapid onset over about 48 h. Progressive facial palsy developing over a period of weeks is usually due either to tumour invading the facial nerve at the skull base (e.g. acoustic neuroma) or within the parotid gland (e.g. adenoid cystic carcinoma). Alternatively it may be due to a demyelinating lesion within the brain.

Action: Refer urgently to neurology or maxillofacial surgery.

9 Inferior alveolar nerve pathology

Unilateral numbness of the lower lip indicates pathology of the inferior alveolar nerve. In the absence of a history of trauma, this mandates urgent investigation. Within the jaw acute osteomyelitis is a benign cause; however, oral squamous cell carcinoma or secondary metastases to the jaw must be excluded. If the jaw is uninvolved, skull base tumours or intracranial tumours or aneurysms are also causes for this symptom, involving the nerve more proximally.

Action: Refer urgently to maxillofacial surgery.

10 Wegener's granulomatosis and midline lethal granuloma

Two life-threatening conditions can affect the hard palate and present with non-healing ulceration. These are Wegener's granulomatosis and midline lethal granuloma, which may be clinically difficult to differentiate. Wegener's is a systemic condition that also affects the lungs and kidneys, whereas midline lethal granuloma is a lymphoma.

Action: Dipstick the urine and do CXR to look for systemic involvement. Refer urgently to maxillofacial surgery.

Orthopaedics

Farhan Ali, Mike Hayton and Gary Miller

1 Acute swelling of a single joint – think of septic arthritis.

2 A painful, swollen finger could be septic flexor tenosynovitis – a surgical emergency.

3 Paediatric trauma may be due to child abuse.

4 An adolescent with a limp, hip or knee pain could have slipped upper femoral epiphysis.

5 Uncontrollable limb pain after injury may be compartment syndrome.

6 Wrist pain after injury – do not miss scaphoid fracture.

7 A skin break overlying any fracture means an open fracture until proved otherwise.

8 A cut on the knuckle is a fight bite until proved otherwise.

9 Not all acute back pains are mechanical.

10 Unexplained bone pain, especially at night, is ominous.

NOTES

1 Septic arthritis

Septic arthritis is serious and difficult to diagnose in the early stages. Typically, the patient presents with fever and an acutely painful, inflamed joint with restricted active and passive range of motion. Atypical presentations can occur in infants and the immunocompromised. Consider the diagnosis in children who refuse to walk or use a limb. In young, sexually active patients with fever and rash, suspect gonococcal arthritis. Antibiotics should be withheld until after joint aspiration and blood cultures are performed. The differential includes crystal disease (gout, pseudogout).

Action: Refer immediately to orthopaedics.

2 Septic flexor tenosynovitis

Flexor tenosynovitis is infection in the flexor sheath, often due to a puncture wound. It is a hand surgery emergency, and so needs to be differentiated from other benign causes of swollen, painful finger. The four cardinal features are: finger held in slight flexion; fusiform swelling of the whole digit; tenderness along the entire flexor tendon sheath; and intense pain with passive extension of the digit. The process can rapidly destroy the flexor tendon sheath and result in loss of function. *Staphylococcus aureus* is the most common organism isolated.

Action: Refer immediately. Keep the patient nil by mouth. Check FBC, ESR, CRP and do blood cultures. Commence IV antibiotics.

3 Child abuse

Failure to recognise child abuse can be ethically and legally catastrophic. In any paediatric trauma, features on history that should raise suspicion include delay in seeking care, implausible or inconsistent history, failure to thrive, prior unusual injury, and repeated accidents, especially if treated at different places. Worrying signs include multiple bruises in infants, head and facial injuries, and cigarette burns. Spiral fractures of the shaft of long bones in children under 2 years, old fractures, rib and skull fractures may have a non-accidental cause. However, differential diagnoses should not be forgotten (coagulopathies, osteogenesis imperfecta, copper deficiency and neuromuscular diseases). The case is handled best by specialists.

Action: Refer immediately to paediatrics with orthopaedic involvement. The child will need a thorough assessment by a clinician experienced in child abuse.

4 Slipped upper femoral epiphysis (SUFE)

SUFE is the most common non-traumatic hip problem in adolescents. Delay in treatment may lead to avascular necrosis of the head of the femur and permanent disability. Diagnosis is often delayed because it can present without hip pain, misleading the unwary. It should be considered in any adolescent with hip, knee or distal thigh pain, limp, or limited range of hip movement. It is more common in overweight, adolescent boys, and is bilateral in about 30%. Presentation is either gradual or acute.

Action: Refer immediately to orthopaedics. In acute cases, do not manipulate the hip, and do not let the patient weight-bear, until assessed by orthopaedics.

5 Compartment syndrome

Fractures and other limb injuries may be complicated by compartment syndrome. This occurs when pressure within closed, fascial compartments exceeds perfusion pressure resulting in muscle ischaemia. The most important feature is unrelenting pain despite opiates, which increases on passive stretch of the fingers or toes whose tendons travel in the compartment(s) affected. The limb may also feel cold, have sensory deficit and be pulseless, but these are often late signs. Causes include trauma, both fractures and soft tissue crush injuries, and constricting casts or bandages. A high index of suspicion is the key to the diagnosis. Surgical fasciotomy may be needed.

Action: Refer immediately to orthopaedics. Keep patient nil by mouth. Split any constricting cast or bandage down to the skin.

6 Scaphoid fracture

A missed scaphoid fracture can lead to long-term patient disability and loss of occupation. It is a common medicolegal case. If there is clinical suspicion due to tenderness over the scaphoid and painful restriction of wrist movement, it is safer to assume that there may be a scaphoid fracture. Initial radiographs may not show evidence of a fracture.

Action: Refer urgently to orthopaedics. Splint the wrist in a backslab while awaiting orthopaedic review.

7 Open fracture

In open fractures, inspection may not reveal exposed bone. A break in the skin near to the fracture could be all there is to see. The most frequent error is to assume the skin disruption does not communicate with the fracture itself. About one-third of patients sustaining an open fracture also have other life-threatening injuries.

Action: Refer immediately to orthopaedics. In the interim, dress the wound, splint the limb and give tetanus prophylaxis. Do not close the wound primarily.

8 Fight bite

A clenched fist injury that results from striking another person's mouth is termed a 'fight bite'. There is typically a small transverse or oblique cut overlying the metacarpophalangeal joint. Though the appearance is deceptively benign, if tooth has penetrated skin, it has also invariably entered the joint capsule. Such injuries require formal debridement by a hand surgeon.

Patients often deny the mechanism of injury so the clinician must have a high index of suspicion.

Action: Refer immediately to orthopaedics. Give appropriate antibiotics. Do not close the wound primarily.

9 Medical causes of acute back pain

Most acute back pain is due to a self-limiting mechanical condition, reflecting degenerative spine processes. However, other serious, medical causes should not be forgotten: dissecting aortic aneurysm, pyelonephritis and ectopic pregnancy.

Action: Consider non-orthopaedic causes of acute back pain.

10 Osteomyelitis and musculoskeletal tumours

Unrelenting bone pain, especially night pain, is ominous. Osteomyelitis is more common in children and often involves the ends of long bones. It often presents with toxaemia, pain and loss of function. However, atypical presentations are not uncommon. Musculoskeletal tumours are rare but can present at any age and can involve any region. Pain is often the first symptom. There may be a firm or ill-defined swelling. Loss of limb function, decreased range of motion or pathological fracture occurs in some patients. Immediate treatment is required for pathological or impending fractures, impending or existing neurological deficits and uncontrollable pain.

Action: Refer urgently to orthopaedics, immediately in situations described above.

Paediatrics

Martha Ford-Adams and Sue Hobbins

1 Beware the baby failing to thrive with absent femoral pulses.

2 Syncope during exercise may be an arrhythmia.

3 Recent onset of cough in a toddler could be due to inhaled foreign body.

4 A baby jaundiced at 2 weeks with pale stools and dark urine needs immediate referral to exclude biliary atresia.

5 A child with bloody diarrhoea or rectal bleeding may have inflammatory bowel disease.

6 A young child who is drinking more and losing weight could be diabetic.

7 Suspect the fat child who is short.

8 Delayed puberty in girls and precocious puberty in boys both need urgent referral.

9 High temperature in a baby under 6 months could be meningitis.

10 The unwell child with a purpuric rash needs antibiotics as an emergency.

11 Back pain in children needs investigating to exclude tumours.

12 Young children who will not walk may have bone or joint infection.

13 Fractures in the non-mobile child are suspicious.

14 Early morning headache and vomiting warrants a brain scan.

15 Coke-coloured brown urine may be nephritis.

NOTES

1 Coarctation of the aorta

Failure to thrive can be assessed by comparing the baby's birth centile to its current centile in the parent-held record. If the current centile is significantly below that at birth, the baby is not thriving. A diagnosis not to miss in these babies is coarctation of the aorta. This is a serious condition that becomes apparent after closure of the ductus arteriosus. Absence of femoral pulses is a reliable sign – they must be palpated in all babies after listening to the heart. Diagnosis is by echocardiogram, and surgery may be required.

Action: Refer urgently.

2 Arrhythmic syncope

Faints are common in young girls, but beware the sudden collapse during exercise. This could be a fit, but arrhythmias secondary to prolonged QT syndrome must be excluded. Prolonged QT syndrome is often undiagnosed and can lead to fatal ventricular tachycardia.

Action: Do an ECG. If the QT interval is greater than 440 ms, refer urgently.

3 Foreign body

Cough is a common complaint in toddlers, usually associated with viral-induced wheeze. Beware the recent onset of cough not preceded by an URTI, and ask parents about possible inhalation of small objects like peanuts, which can get stuck in the right main bronchus. Bronchoscopy may be needed.

Action: Do a CXR. (The child will not be cooperative enough for inspiratory and expiratory films at this stage.) If collapse is seen, refer immediately.

4 Biliary atresia

Biliary atresia is a rare but significant cause of prolonged jaundice (over 2 weeks) in the neonatal period. It needs urgent treatment to relieve the obstruction otherwise liver failure ensues, so early detection is vital. Pale stools and dark urine are signs indicating biliary obstruction. Dark-skinned babies do not look as jaundiced as light-skinned babies – inspecting the sclerae can be helpful. A split bilirubin to determine the amount that is conjugated, and ultrasound to assess the biliary tree, are needed to make the diagnosis.

Action: If jaundice is present beyond 2 weeks of age, refer immediately. If in doubt about the presence of jaundice, refer anyway for serum bilirubin.

5 Inflammatory bowel disease

Bloody diarrhoea is rare in children. Once infectious causes have been excluded, inflammatory bowel disease needs to be considered, especially if patient is not gaining weight.

Action: Check weight and height. Arrange stool culture. Check ESR, CRP and serum albumin. Refer urgently.

6 Diabetes

The incidence of type 1 diabetes in children under 5 years has doubled recently. As these children are often in nappies, it can be difficult to detect polyuria, leading to delay in diagnosis. As a result, they are more likely to be acidotic and dehydrated at diagnosis. Together with their relatively greater cerebral mass, this increases the risk of potentially fatal cerebral oedema. Diabetes should be considered in any toddler who has lost weight and is drinking more than normal. Glycosuria in children is always significant.

Action: Dipstick the urine in the nappy. If there is glycosuria, refer immediately.

7 Obesity

Obesity is increasing in children due to higher calorie intake and decreased exercise. Obese children are nearly always tall for their age. Overweight children who are short, however, may have an endocrine cause for their growth failure.

Action: Plot the child on a growth chart or ask if he is the tallest in the class. If the child is short (for parents, in his class, or below the 3rd centile), refer. All other obese children just need a diet!

8 Puberty

The age of puberty is falling in girls but the trend is not so apparent in boys. If a boy is growing rapidly and has testicular or genital enlargement before 9 years of age, he needs urgent referral to exclude congenital adrenal hyperplasia or testicular tumour. A girl with delayed puberty needs referral for a karyotype to exclude Turner's syndrome.

Action: If a boy is growing rapidly, examine his testicles and genitalia to assess pubertal stage and refer urgently. Refer urgently a girl with delayed puberty.

9 Meningitis

Temperature is a common complaint in infants but is often not assessed accurately by parents. It is vital to measure it, as it can be the only sign of meningitis in this age group. Other signs like neck stiffness, irritability or headache are rare at this age and the baby can look deceptively well.

Action: Measure the temperature of babies. If $> 38°C$, refer immediately.

10 Meningococcal sepsis

Meningococcal sepsis is rare, but rapidly fatal in children. It presents with a non-blanching, purpuric rash in an unwell, usually pyrexial, child. The priority is to start antibiotics.

Microbiological cultures can be taken later and initial treatment with penicillin will not affect the child.

Action: Give IM penicillin immediately. Refer immediately.

11 Spinal tumours

Unlike headaches and abdominal pain, back pain is rare in children. Mobility may be restricted when children bend down (the mini-skirt sign). It is important to exclude tumours in these children (solid or leukaemic deposits).

Action: Refer urgently.

12 Orthopaedic infection

Refusal to walk or use a limb is an unusual symptom and septic arthritis or oesteomyelitis need to be excluded even if the child is relatively well. Alternatively, the child may have sustained a fracture unknown to parents.

Action: Refer urgently to orthopaedics.

13 Non-accidental injury

It is rare for non-mobile children to sustain fractures. As a result, there should be concern as to whether the accident was truly accidental.

Action: Document the history in detail at the outset – in child protection cases, histories often change over time. Refer urgently.

14 Brain tumour

Headaches are a very common complaint in children. However, if worse in the morning, especially if associated with vomiting, a brain tumour needs to be excluded by imaging.

Action: Refer urgently.

15 Nephritis

Acute post-streptococcal nephritis presents with haematuria (urine looks like coke) and oliguria. These signs can be subtle in children who are not keen to show their urine and the brown discoloration is often not considered serious. These children can progress to renal failure quickly and need admission.

Action: Refer 'brown' urine immediately.

Paediatric surgery

Mark Davenport and Stein Erik Haugen

1 A tender groin, scrotal or labial swelling could be an incarcerated inguinal hernia.

2 Infants with attacks of persistent screaming may have intussusception.

3 Bile-stained vomiting – think of surgical causes.

4 Bile-stained vomiting with abdominal tenderness in an unwell infant may herald life-threatening volvulus.

5 Non-bilious, persistent vomiting in an infant 2–8 weeks old could be pyloric stenosis.

6 Frothy saliva at a neonate's mouth means oesophageal atresia until proved otherwise.

7 Coughing and spluttering during feeding, and recurrent pneumonia, can be caused by tracheo-oesophageal fistula.

8 'Gastroenteritis' in a young child could be appendicitis.

9 Bilateral undescended, impalpable testes with an abnormal phallus – do not miss congenital adrenal hyperplasia.

NOTES

1 Incarcerated inguinal hernia

Most inguinal hernias in children are reducible and non-tender. Incarceration is not uncommon, however, especially in infants. If they become tender and painful, and are difficult to reduce, incarcerated intestine, testis or ovary is at risk of ischaemic damage. A small proportion of boys diagnosed with hydrocele will actually have an incomplete inguinal hernial sac within the inguinal canal, and this may become irreducible and therefore painful.

Action: Refer immediately to paediatric surgery.

2 Intussusception

Most infants will have simple colic at some point in the first year of life. Sudden onset of persistent screaming, pulling legs up and refusing feeds or vomiting in an older infant (7–10 months) should raise suspicion of an intussusception. This is the commonest cause of acute abdominal pain requiring intervention in children under 3 years. A mass in the upper abdomen may be palpable in the infant's quieter moments and is diagnostic.

Action: Refer immediately to paediatric surgery. Consider IV fluids if clinically dehydrated.

3 Acute volvulus

If the fetal bowel fails to rotate and fixate normally, intestinal mobility is increased and there is risk of midgut volvulus. This can lead to intestinal obstruction with ischaemia of the twisted gut. Without immediate surgery, this rapidly progresses to bowel gangrene, resulting in death or loss of the entire small intestine. It is therefore a true surgical emergency. Onset of bilious vomiting in a previously well baby is the main presenting symptom, accompanied by generalised abdominal pain, deterioration of the general condition and sometimes passage of blood per rectum.

Action: Refer immediately to paediatric surgery. Give IV fluids.

4 Bowel obstruction

Vomiting is common throughout childhood, but is usually gastric contents alone. The presence of bile (which should always be confirmed with parents as 'green bile', rather than simply the sour taste of refluxed gastric acid) is indicative of a more distal mechanical obstruction. The causes tend to vary with the age of the child. For instance, in neonates this may indicate a duodenal atresia, a malrotation or a small bowel atresia. In an older infant, intussusception or an obstructed hernia should be looked for.

Action: Refer immediately to paediatric surgery. Consider IV fluids if clinically dehydrated.

5 Hypertrophic pyloric stenosis

Hypertrophic pyloric stenosis is a common cause of gastric outlet obstruction in infants a few weeks old. Non-bilious vomiting starts off infrequently and becomes progressively more frequent and forceful. A delay in diagnosis and treatment will lead to significant dehydration and lethargy.

Action: Refer urgently to paediatric surgery.

6. Oesophageal atresia

Inability of a newborn to swallow its own saliva must be assumed to be due to oeosphageal atresia until proved otherwise. The attempted passage of a fair-sized nasogastric tube (e.g. 8 Fg) and a CXR will clarify whether the oesophagus is patent.

Action: Refer immediately to paediatrics.

7 Tracheo-oesophageal fistula

Congenital, isolated tracheo-oesophageal fistula is an uncommon variant within the spectrum of oesophageal atresia. It can remain undiagnosed for a prolonged period of time, causing considerable morbidity and sometimes lung damage. It should be considered in cases of recurrent pneumonia, or when coughing and spluttering interrupt feeds.

Action: Refer urgently to paediatric surgery.

8 Acute appendicitis

In children below 4 years, appendicitis is a rare cause of acute abdominal pain, and the presentation tends to be different compared with older children. It regularly mimics gastroenteritis with vomiting, diarrhoea and high fever accompanying the pain. This often leads to a delay in surgical referral, and the perforation rate is high. Have a low threshold for a surgical opinion in a young child with acute abdominal pain and tenderness.

Action: Refer immediately to paediatric surgery.

9 Congenital adrenal hyperplasia

Bilateral undescended (and impalpable) 'testes', and perhaps a smaller-than-normal phallus, may indicate ambiguous genitalia. One cause of this, congenital adrenal hyperplasia, may have profound electrolyte abnormalities (hyponatraemia) leading to sudden collapse and shock. These children are genetically female, although the genitalia are virilised, with labia resembling scrotal tissue, and clitoral hypertrophy. Checking electrolytes will resolve whether there is an associated mineralocorticoid deficit, needing hormone replacement and IV saline.

Action: Refer urgently to paediatrics.

Plastic surgery

Sarah Pape, Navin Singh and Paul Manson

1 Hoarse voice after burn injury – airway is at risk.

2 Facial muscle stiffness following a recent wound may be tetanus.

3 Light-headedness and racing heartbeat after a scalp laceration – think of blood loss.

4 A sick, pyrexial patient with cellulitis could have life-threatening necrotising fasciitis.

5 An unwell, feverish child with a minor burn could have toxic shock syndrome.

6 Numbness, tingling, weakness or poor circulation after a penetrating wound suggest nerve, tendon or vessel injury.

7 Following surgery under local anaesthesia, perioral tingling, metallic taste and confusion may signal lidocaine toxicity.

8 A painful, swollen stiff digit or hand after a high-pressure injection injury needs urgent exploration.

9 Cellulitis after a cut in an aquatic environment can be devastating.

10 Malocclusion of teeth after facial trauma – suspect facial fracture.

NOTES

1 Airway burn

Hoarseness of the voice is an early symptom of laryngeal oedema. If the hoarseness is ignored, complete upper airway obstruction may follow. Patients with facial burns have a high incidence of airway burns due to the inhalation of hot gas or liquid. Closed space burns (car fire, house fire) are high risk for smoke inhalation. Associated signs include singed nasal hairs and carbonaceous sputum. Treatment is immediate control of the airway with prophylactic intubation while still feasible.

Action: Administer humidified, high-flow oxygen through a facemask with a reservoir bag. Refer immediately to the emergency department for the attention of a senior anaesthetist.

2 Tetanus

Stiffness of facial, especially jaw, muscles is an early symptom of tetanus ('lockjaw'). In the developed world, the symptoms may be mild due to partial immunity. They come on 2–20 days after skin injury from a wound, burn or surgery, often associated with dirt, debris or agrarian environments. Full-blown tetanus progresses from facial stiffness to spasticity of skeletal muscles, accompanied by dysphagia, neck stiffness, rigidity of the abdominal muscles and difficulty in breathing. The patient may develop painful muscle spasms provoked by touch, sound, light or emotion. Consciousness is not impaired. Autonomic symptoms include tachycardia, tachypnoea, profuse sweating and cardiovascular collapse, which may be sudden and fatal.

Action: Refer immediately to an intensive care unit (ICU). Give IM human tetanus immunoglobulin and antitetanus toxoid (at different sites).

3 Blood loss from scalp laceration

A scalp laceration can often have significant associated blood loss. As much as 1–2 units of blood can be lost at the site of a large scalp laceration, and more is lost during transport and evaluation at the emergency department. Light-headedness or postural hypotension may indicate hypovolaemic shock and blood-loss anaemia. With significant head trauma and intracranial injury, the hypotension may be due to neurogenic shock, but this is usually rare.

Action: Check pulse and BP (lying and standing). Check FBC. Replace fluids and transfuse if necessary.

4 Necrotising fasciitis

Necrotising fasciitis usually has an insidious onset, with localised pain and swelling of the soft tissues, followed by mild cellulitis of the overlying skin. It is commoner in older people, diabetics and intravenous drug users. Infection of the soft tissue spreads along fascial planes over a few hours or days. Muscle necrosis may occur. The patient becomes increasingly unwell, with fever, malaise and cardiovascular collapse. The mortality rate is 50%. The infection is usually due to a combination of a Gram-positive coccus and a Gram-negative bacillus. The early stages of the disease may be indistinguishable from gas gangrene. The patient needs early, radical excision of all the necrotic tissues. If the patient survives, he or she may require major reconstructive surgery.

Action: Refer immediately to plastic surgery in a hospital with an ICU. Commence IV fluids and give high-dose, broad-spectrum antibiotics intravenously. If gas gangrene is suspected, include high-dose penicillin.

5 Toxic shock syndrome

Many young children with minor burns have low-grade pyrexia and feel generally unwell and grumpy. These symptoms alone are not a cause for concern. However, such children can deteriorate very rapidly with high fever, lethargy, diarrhoea, vomiting, diffuse macular rash and cardiovascular collapse. The usual cause is a toxin-producing *Staphylococcus aureus*.

Action: Refer immediately to a paediatric burn centre or paediatric ICU. Commence IV or intra-osseous fluid resuscitation and IV antibiotics (flucloxacillin or clindamycin). Give fresh frozen plasma (FFP) (it contains the antistaphylococcal antibodies that the child lacks).

6 Penetrating injury

Numbness, tingling, weakness or poor circulation after a penetrating wound suggests that there is injury to nerves, tendons or vessels. Children and intoxicated patients may not be able to describe these symptoms clearly, so have a high degree of suspicion. A spike of glass can cause a minor skin wound with severe disruption to deeper structures. Incomplete nerve injuries may produce a confusing pattern of sensory and motor loss. All penetrating wounds with sensory, circulatory or motor loss need to be surgically explored.

Action: Refer immediately to a hand surgeon or to plastic surgery.

7 Lidocaine toxicity

Lidocaine (lignocaine) is used as a local anaesthetic in a wide variety of procedures in outpatient and primary care settings. Toxicity is rare but potentially fatal. Early symptoms include perioral tingling, metallic taste in the mouth, and confusion or agitation. This may proceed to seizures, cardiac arrythmias and death. Treatment involves benzodiazepines to lower seizure potential, possible intubation, and intensive care.

Action: Refer immediately to the emergency department.

8 High-pressure injection injury

High-pressure injection of air, oil or paint into a digit may cause a trivial entry wound but lead to severe disability and amputation. The point of entry is usually the tip of the thumb or index finger of the non-dominant hand. The wound feels a little uncomfortable at first but becomes increasingly painful over a few hours. The injected substance tracks through the tissue planes and causes fat necrosis. X-rays may reveal air or radio-opaque material in the soft tissues. Early, radical debridement, with possible amputation and reconstruction, may be necessary.

Action: Refer immediately to a hand surgeon.

9 Cellulitis from aquatic organisms

Even relatively innocuous scrapes or cuts in an aquatic environment can develop aggressive infections that need treatment with operative debridement and IV antibiotics. *Vibrio vulnificus* is an aggressive, life-threatening organism responsible for such infections.

Action: Refer immediately to plastic surgery.

10 Malocclusion after facial trauma

Malocclusion of the teeth after facial trauma is a very sensitive symptom of maxillary or mandibular fractures. CT scanning is used for evaluation.

Action: Refer urgently to plastic or maxillofacial surgery.

Psychiatry

Niruj Agrawal and Steven Hirsch

1 Sudden onset of fluctuating disorientation is a feature of delirium.

2 Decline in functioning in older people could be due to dementia.

3 Never forget to ask about ideas of self-harm from a psychiatric or depressed patient.

4 Agitation, with muscular tension or threats, often precedes violence.

5 Do not miss depression in a general hospital setting.

6 A young person behaving oddly with change in personality may have a psychotic illness.

7 Racing thoughts and overactivity suggest a manic illness.

8 Eager dieting in a thin girl with amenorrhoea – think of anorexia nervosa.

9 Palpitations or faintness in a young person could be anxiety disorder.

10 Acute alcohol withdrawal can cause serious neurological problems.

NOTES

1 Delirium (acute confusional state)

A sudden onset of disorientation with fluctuating conscious-ness is a common presentation of delirium. Perceptual disturb-ances and agitation may also occur. When the presentation includes prominent delusions, hallucinations and behavioural problems, it may be mistaken for a psychotic illness. Fluctuating cognitive impairment always needs investigation. Possible causes include medications, infection, metabolic or neurological disease, and withdrawal from alcohol or drugs. Delay in diagnosis and treatment can be fatal. Management is directed towards diagnosing and treating the underlying cause of delir-ium while providing good supportive care and sedation.

Action: Refer immediately to medical admissions. If the differ-ential diagnosis of psychosis is being considered, request a psychiatric opinion.

2 Dementia

Gradual decline in personal and social functioning in older individuals could be an early manifestation of dementia. Early presentations may include depression or psychotic features. Conversely, depression or other psychiatric illnesses may mimic dementia. It is also important to rule out other neurological problems such as a space-occupying lesion, metabolic causes, head injury and stroke.

Action: Take a detailed history including an independent account from a relative. Perform a neurological examination and mental state examination with special emphasis on higher brain functions. Always test recall of recent and remote memory. Refer to the old age psychiatry team at an early stage.

3 Suicide

Suicide is a common and often preventable complication of psychiatric illnesses. Assessment of any psychiatric or de-pressed patient should always include enquiry of any ideas, plan or intent of deliberate self-harm. This is particularly important in people who have past history of self-harm or those with evidence of depression. Contrary to common belief, asking about suicidal ideas does not increase suicide risk.

Action: Urgently refer to psychiatry any patient with suicidal ideas or plans. Document mental state examination and risk assessment.

4 Violence

Most violent individuals in our society are not mentally ill or definable as patients. Violence in medical settings could be due to a neurological or organic disorder, drug or alcohol intoxication, or a diagnosable psychiatric disorder. Early recognition of signs of imminent violence like agitation, muscular tension or threats may help in prevention or in decreasing risk of injury to staff or patients. Past history of violence is the most reliable predictor of the current potential of violence.

Action: Consider the safety of staff and other patients first. Call security if necessary. Management includes de-escalation strategies and sedation. Urgently seek a psychiatric opinion if evidence of psychiatric illness is present.

5 Depression in a general hospital setting

Depression is a very common comorbidity in hospital patients with acute or chronic medical and surgical problems. It is under-recognised and results in poor compliance and outcome, inappropriate investigations and prolonged and frequent admissions. Characteristic features include sustained depressed mood, anhedonia (loss of ability to experience pleasure), social withdrawal and depressive cognitions like guilt and hopelessness.

Action: Obtain a detailed psychosocial history and speak to family members. If concerned, request an opinion from a liaison psychiatrist.

6 Psychotic illness

A young person presenting with gradual or sudden change in personality or social functioning, along with strange or odd behaviour, may have a psychotic illness like schizophrenia. Also consider other cerebral pathology and illicit drug use.

Action: Perform a detailed mental state examination including enquiry into abnormal perceptions and beliefs. Refer urgently to psychiatry.

7 Bipolar disorder

Manic episodes, as part of a bipolar disorder, commonly manifest with racing thoughts, overactivity, impulsivity, disinhibition and sometimes grandiose delusions. The individual may be at risk of financial and sexual exploitation. Untreated, a prolonged and severe manic episode may develop, leading to exhaustion and risk to life.

Action: Refer urgently to psychiatry. Admission or assessment under the Mental Health Act may be required.

8 Anorexia nervosa

Always think of anorexia nervosa in a thin young girl eager to lose weight. Primary or secondary amenorrhoea is a diagnostic feature. Features to look for include excessive dieting, induced vomiting or laxative abuse. A characteristic feature is self-perception of being overweight despite being thin and underweight (body image disturbance). Anorexia nervosa, if left untreated, results in metabolic and endocrinal complications, and can be life-threatening. Bulimia nervosa involves binging and vomiting to maintain normal weight.

Action: Measure height and weight and calculate body mass index (BMI = weight (kg)/height (m^2)) and inquire about body image disturbance. Refer urgently to psychiatry.

9 Anxiety disorders

Episodes of sudden onset of palpitation, faintness and hyper-ventilation are common manifestation of anxiety disorders, such as panic attacks. Often patients presenting with these features are referred to cardiology, neurology or other medical specialities, and undergo unnecessary investigations.

Action: Refer to psychiatry if an organic condition seems unlikely.

10 Acute alcohol withdrawal

Acute withdrawal of alcohol in a patient dependent on alcohol can result in disabling, life-threatening, neurological complications. These can be prevented, however. They include delirium tremens and Wernicke's encephalopathy, which are medical emergencies. The early features of acute withdrawal include anxiety, insomnia, tremor and sweats. Fits may also develop.

Action: Refer immediately to medical admissions. Monitor the patient carefully for neurological complications, looking especially for nystagmus, ophthalmoplegia and ataxia. Give benzodiazepines, titrating the dose carefully. Administer thiamine parenterally without delay, and ensure adequate hydration. In presence of neurological signs above, request an immediate neurological opinion.

Renal medicine

Andrew Fry and John Bradley

---

1 New visual symptoms could be severe hypertension.

2 New onset of oedema may be due to protein loss in the urine.

3 A UTI in a child is worrying – think of a structural abnormality.

4 With complex symptoms always ask: could this be vasculitis?

5 Always test for haematuria in a patient with haemoptysis.

6 Not all hypertension is essential – there may be a treatable, renal cause.

7 Malaise and itch may indicate renal failure.

8 Cloudy dialysate bags warn of peritonitis.

9 When a fistula thrill stops, thrombosis must be urgently excluded.

NOTES

1 Severe hypertension

Severe hypertension (diastolic BP > 120 mmHg) may present with visual disturbance caused by retinopathy. As a result, measurement of BP should be part of the assessment of the patient presenting with new visual symptoms.

Action: Check for retinal haemorrhages and papilloedema, if possible. Refer immediately to medicine.

2 Nephrotic syndrome

Although oedema has many causes, the appearance of a new onset of oedema, especially if generalised or in the presence of other systemic symptoms, should alert one to the potential for renal disease. If there is significant proteinuria on dipstick testing, nephrotic syndrome is the likely underlying cause.

Action: Dipstick the urine, check the BP and U&E arrange for a 24-h urine collection to quantify proteinuria. Discuss with the renal unit about further investigation.

3 Childhood UTIs

All children with even a single UTI, confirmed microbiologically, should be investigated to exclude the presence of renal tract structural abnormalities and vesico-ureteric reflux. Undetected, these can lead to the development of chronic renal failure in later years. Remember, UTIs in children can present without the classic symptoms of dysuria, loin pain and frequency. Non-specific symptoms, such as fever, vomiting and lethargy, may be the only clues.

Action: Culture the urine, treat with appropriate antibiotics and refer to paediatrics for further assessment.

4 Vasculitis

Vasculitis should be considered in the differential diagnosis of patients presenting with a complex assortment of symptoms. Other suggestive features include systemic symptoms (e.g. fever, malaise, weight loss), skin changes (pupuric, erythematous or netlike rash) and abnormal urinalysis and renal function.

Action: Dipstick the urine, check U&E, LFTs, FBC, ESR, CRP, clotting screen, autoantibodies and antineutrophil cytoplasmic antibody (ANCA) (if present, confirms systemic vasculitis). Refer to medicine, rheumatology or, if renal involvement, to nephrology.

5 Pulmonary–renal syndromes

Although haemoptysis has many causes, it can be a presenting feature of conditions with both lung and kidney involvement, such as small-vessel vasculitis and antiglomerular basement membrane (Goodpasture's) disease. As a result, urinalysis for haematuria is mandatory on all patients who cough up blood. Prompt treatment is required to preserve renal function and save life.

Action: Dipstick the urine. If positive for blood, do urgent urine microscopy (looking for casts) and U&E. Refer immediately to nephrology.

6 Renal causes of hypertension

Urine dipstick testing must be a routine part of the assessment of any person newly presenting with hypertension. The finding of blood and/or protein may imply the presence of a renal cause, which may be treatable.

Action: Dipstick the urine. If positive for blood and/or protein, send the urine for microscopy and culture (to exclude an infective cause), and check U&E. Refer to nephrology.

7 Chronic renal failure

Unfortunately, chronic renal impairment tends not to present with any clear-cut symptoms. Most patients just feel generally 'under the weather' and there is little to suggest the diagnosis. Pruritus is often a feature of end-stage disease and may be secondary to abnormal calcium and phosphate metabolism. Have a higher index of suspicion in those patients who may have risk factors for renal disease – such as hypertension or diabetes (although the renal function of these patients should be under monitoring anyway) – or if there is a family history.

Action: Check U&E.

8 Peritoneal dialysis (PD) peritonitis

PD involves the exchange of volumes of dialysis fluid into and out of the peritoneal cavity a number of times each day. Peritonitis is the most important complication and the first sign is often cloudiness of the 'drained-out' dialysis fluid. Abdominal symptoms and signs, plus systemic upset, may also coexist. Prompt treatment with appropriate antibiotics is vital to prevent later complications.

Action: Refer immediately to the local renal centre – the patient should have a contact number for the PD nursing team.

9 Fistula thrombosis

Arteriovenous fistulae are the preferred form of vascular access for haemodialysis patients. A thrill is present at the anastomotic site and patients should monitor this. If it stops, a thrombosis should be suspected and urgent assessment is required.

Action: Refer urgently to the renal unit.

Respiratory medicine

Chris Stenton and Jeremy George

1 Haemoptysis should be investigated in smokers over 40.

2 Do not ignore shoulder pain in smokers over 40.

3 Weight loss and night sweats may be due to tuberculosis.

4 Falling asleep while driving or at work may be due to obstructive sleep apnoea.

5 Not all wheezing is caused by asthma.

6 An asthmatic who wakes at night with cough and wheeze is at risk of a life-threatening attack.

7 Early morning headache in a patient with lung disease may be due to carbon dioxide retention.

8 A stuffy nose with chest symptoms could indicate Wegener's granulomatosis.

9 Do not forget to ask about the budgie!

10 An asthmatic with nasal polyps might be hypersensitive to NSAIDs.

NOTES

1 Haemoptysis

Coughing up blood is an alarming symptom but does not necessarily imply serious underlying lung disease. It can be difficult, therefore, to know how extensively to investigate the patient. In a patient at low risk for lung cancer, with isolated haemoptysis, no further action is usually required if the CXR is normal. Conversely, further investigation is needed in smokers over the age of 40, as approximately 2% will be found to have a tumour.

Repeated haemoptysis should always be investigated regardless of the CXR findings and risk factors for lung cancer. Although rare, non-smokers may develop lung tumours. Other possible diagnoses include bronchiectasis, which can be difficult to detect on a CXR, and pulmonary embolism, particularly following immobilisation or recent travel.

Action: Arrange urgent CXR. Refer to the chest clinic, urgently in smokers over 40.

2 Pancoast's tumour

Tumours arising from the apex of the lung may grow into the chest wall and brachial plexus, and are known as Pancoast's tumours. They characteristically cause excruciating pain in the shoulder and inner aspect of the arm but may be mistaken for minor shoulder conditions. Other features of Pancoast's tumours are Horner's syndrome, loss of sensation in the T1 dermatome and weakness of the small muscles of the hand. Pancoast's tumours are easily missed on plain X-rays and the patient should still be referred if clinical suspicion persists.

Action: Examine for the features above and arrange urgent CXR. Refer urgently to the chest clinic.

3 Tuberculosis

TB is becoming increasingly common both worldwide and in the UK. Individuals at particular risk include immigrants from countries where the disease is endemic, alcoholics, patients with HIV and healthcare workers. A history of weight loss and night sweats may indicate active disease. Productive and persistent cough is the commonest respiratory symptom.

Action: Ask about risk factors and possible TB contacts. Arrange CXR, and check FBC, ESR and CRP. Refer to a TB clinic directly if the CXR is suggestive of TB. If uncertain, refer to a chest clinic, as other possibilities, such as lymphoma, may need to be excluded.

4 Obstructive sleep apnoea

Obstructive sleep apnoea classically affects middle-aged, overweight men with short necks. Their partners may complain that they snore loudly and they may even notice that they develop apnoeic episodes while asleep. As a result of their poor quality of sleep, they may have trouble concentrating during the day and may even fall asleep at work. This may have profound effects on their professional and personal lives and can result in tragedy if they fall asleep while driving or operating machinery.

Action: Refer to a sleep clinic. Offer advice to lose weight (if appropriate) and to avoid drinking alcohol or taking a sedative at night. Advise not to drive or work with machinery if there is a risk of falling asleep.

5 Non-asthmatic wheeze

The diagnosis of asthma is usually clinical and based on relatively non-specific symptoms. However, other organic diseases (e.g. lung cancer, chronic obstructive pulmonary disease (COPD), cardiac failure and some laryngeal conditions) may mimic asthma by causing breathlessness and wheeze. In addition, psychogenic conditions, associated with hyperventilation and disproportionate breathlessness, may also be mistaken for asthma. None of these respond to standard asthma treatment and failure to improve should prompt a search for an alternative or additional diagnosis.

Action: Reconsider the diagnosis in an 'asthmatic' who fails to respond to treatment.

6 Uncontrolled asthma

Young asthmatics are more likely to have brittle disease and to ignore their symptoms, with tragic consequences. A history of waking at night with cough and wheeze is an important indicator of poorly controlled asthma. Many asthmatics are reluctant to take inhaled corticosteroids and rely exclusively on their bronchodilators. They may obtain temporary relief before going to bed but wake a few hours later with very severe bronchospasm.

Action: Refer urgently to the chest clinic. Emphasise the importance of taking steroid inhalers regularly. If the patient is severely breathless and wheezy, refer immediately to casualty.

7 Carbon dioxide retention

Carbon dioxide retention may develop insidiously and can be easily overlooked. It is important to diagnose as it may lead to narcosis and death. Characteristically, patients complain of severe headaches on waking in the morning. Patients at risk include those with COPD (who may be on long-term oxygen therapy) and those with severe kyphoscoliotic deformities and neuromuscular disease. This latter group may also report breathlessness on lying flat.

Action: Refer urgently to the chest clinic or to a dedicated sleep clinic.

8 Wegener's granulomatosis

Wegener's granulomatosis is an uncommon necrotising vasculitis that affects particularly the upper airways, lungs and kidneys. The upper airway symptoms may be minor and mentioned only as an afterthought, as patients concentrate on the cough, haemoptysis and symptoms associated with renal disease or cutaneous vasculitis. Symptoms of nasal stuffiness should not be overlooked as they may provide a clue to diagnosing this otherwise elusive multisystem disease. The diagnosis is usually established from the presence of characteristic antibodies in the blood.

Action: Check serum antineutrophil cytoplasmic antibody (ANCA). Refer urgently to the chest clinic.

9 Extrinsic allergic bronchiolo-alveolitis

Extrinsic allergic bronchiolo-alveolitis is most easily identified from the acute flulike symptoms that develop a few hours after exposure when individuals have intermittent contact with the causative agent. Patients who live with a budgerigar at home tend to have chronic low-level exposures and can develop more insidious pulmonary fibrosis without obvious acute episodes – the chronic form of the disease. Breathlessness is accompanied by absent or few physical signs. Finger clubbing is rare. The diagnosis can usually be established from serum IgG antibodies (precipitins) and CT abnormalities, but will be missed unless the pets are enquired about.

Action: Check serum avian precipitins. Refer to the chest clinic.

10 Aspirin-sensitive asthma

About 2% of asthmatics report some degree of aspirin sensitivity. It is more common in women, those with adult onset of disease and those with severe unstable asthma. The response to ingesting aspirin or other NSAIDs can be dramatic, with life-threatening bronchoconstriction developing within minutes. About 60% of patients with aspirin-sensitive asthma have nasal polyps. Caution should therefore be exercised in prescribing NSAIDs to an asthmatic with this finding. Aspirin and other NSAIDs should be avoided completely if there is a history of a previous adverse reaction.

Action: Avoid prescribing aspirin and other NSAIDs to asthmatics with nasal polyps or a history of previous adverse reactions.

Rheumatology

Paul Emery, Lori Siegel and Robert Sanders

1 A young female with a rash may have lupus.

2 Attempted suicide could be a complication of lupus or its treatment.

3 A young person with acute arthritis may have sarcoidosis.

4 Not everyone with a stiff neck and a high ESR has polymyalgia.

5 A patient who becomes unwell after reducing steroids may have life-threatening Addisonian crisis.

6 Thigh or groin pain could have a spinal nerve root origin.

7 Not all swollen ankles are due to heart failure.

8 A rheumatoid patient who goes 'off legs' may be at risk of spinal cord compression.

9 Joint pains in a healthy young adult could be Lyme disease.

10 A young patient with back pain and stiffness could have ankylosing spondylitis.

NOTES

1 Systemic lupus erythematosus (SLE) – skin

SLE is an autoimmune disease with a vast array of manifestations. Beware the young female with a rash (especially a
photosensitive one) until lupus has been excluded. A common
scenario is a young girl presenting with history of reddening
in the sun or with a slight rash. These patients may well
have early lupus, and for them certain therapies including
the contraceptive pill will be contraindicated. The presence of
livedo reticularis (a netlike rash) is an important clue to the
presence of anticardolipin antibody.

Action: Refer to rheumatology or dermatology.

2 SLE – psychosis

Approximately two-thirds of SLE patients suffer neuropsy-
chiatric symptoms including mood disorders, anxiety and
frank psychosis. In addition, exacerbations of SLE are often
treated with high-dose steroids, which may precipitate frank
psychosis. These psychotic patients are at increased risk of
personal injury and suicide.

Action: Refer immediately to psychiatry.

3 Sarcoidosis

Arthritis lasting a few days to 3 months occurs in 10–15% of
patients with sarcoidosis. The arthritis can be of sudden
onset, unilateral or symmetrical, often involving the feet and
ankles. Axial skeleton sparing, with 2–6 joints affected, and
periarticular pain far greater than objective signs would suggest are suspicious for sarcoidosis. Prevalence is higher in
those aged between 20 and 30 years, especially in patients
of Afro-Caribbean descent. Biopsy is positive in over 90%.
Corticosteroids may help control acute symptoms, and can be
tapered after the addition of a disease-modifying agent.
The long-term goal is to prevent late sequelae including cor
pulmonale.

Action: Do CXR, serum ACE (high) and calcium (high). Refer to rheumatology and other appropriate specialities.

4 Neck pain and high ESR

Neck pain is a very common symptom, and high ESR also has many causes. For example, a patient with cervical spondylosis and hyperlipidemia will have neck pain (often with stiffness) as well as high ESR, and may appear to respond to a small dose of steroids. As a result, do not assume that all patients with an elevated ESR and stiffness in the neck have polymyalgia. Furthermore, small doses of steroids can often help osteoarthritis, apparently confirming the incorrect diagnosis. It is not uncommon, therefore, for patients to receive long-term steroids inappropriately for osteoarthritis. When in doubt, a simple way of confirming that high ESR is due to inflammation is to check the CRP.

Action: Check CRP along with ESR.

5 Addisonian crisis

Addisonian crisis, with nausea, vomiting, fever, hyperkalemia, hypoglycemia and/or hyponatremia, with or without an exacerbation of the underlying inflammatory process, is typical of acute steroid withdrawal. This withdrawal syndrome may be life-threatening and should be picked up quickly. A slow, careful taper taking weeks to months is recommended for any long-term use of systemic corticosteroids. Such taper is advised even if dosing is as low as 5 mg per day (physiologic range). Patient education is essential for compliance and safety. Patients should wear a medic alert bracelet, or carry a steroid card, if on corticosteroids more than 5 mg for 10 days in the previous year.

Action: Refer immediately to medical admissions.

6 Femoral nerve root compression

Always remember to do the femoral nerve stretch test. Sciatica is rarely missed by primary care physicians, but femoral nerve involvement is. Whenever there is pain in the groin or thigh, relieved by bending forward, or exacerbated when going downstairs, consider involvement of the higher lumbar roots. Trapping at this site will give a positive femoral nerve stretch test, elicited by lying the patient face down on a couch. There may be other neurological involvement such as reduced knee reflex. Therapy aims to relieve pressure on the nerve root.

Action: Check femoral nerve stretch test and knee reflex if suspected from history. Refer to orthopaedics or rheumatology.

7 Ruptured Baker's cyst

Swollen ankles are not always due to heart failure. Patients with a knee effusion or ruptured Baker's cyst can develop ankle oedema. When the ruptured effusions are bilateral, it can be very misleading unless a careful history has been taken. Diuretics should not be the automatic response to swollen ankles.

Action: Ask about history of swollen joint. If present, refer to rheumatology.

8 Rheumatoid and 'off legs'

In a patient with known rheumatoid disease who goes 'off legs', worsening arthritis should not be assumed to be the cause. The situation is frequently due to one of the following two conditions: atlantoaxial subluxation in the cervical spine, which can cause signs of cord compression; or more commonly, pelvic insufficiency fracture, which causes severe pain on weight-bearing but is relieved after lying flat. The correct diagnosis is vital because the conditions are treated in quite different ways.

Action: Refer immediately to rheumatology or neurology.

9 Lyme disease

While Lyme arthritis itself is neither an acute nor a life-threatening condition, failure to diagnose it early may result in debilitating sequelae: involvement of the CNS and heart. In any person (especially young or previously healthy) complaining of joint pains without an obvious cause, Lyme disease should be considered. Ask about prior tick bite (recalled in only 30%), rash (erythema migrans), or travel to endemic regions (north-eastern and upper mid-western areas of USA). Early antibiotic therapy is curative.

Action: Check serology and/or PCR for the causative agent, *Borrelia burgdorferi*.

10 Ankylosing spondylitis

The diagnosis of ankylosing spondylitis is often delayed for more than 10 years as, in the early stages, the pain responds to NSAIDs and radiographs are normal. In patients with back pain associated with early morning stiffness, particularly if the onset is insidious before age 40 years, persistent for more than 3 months, and relieved by exercise or worsened by rest, ankylosing spondylitis should be considered. The condition is treatable if diagnosed early enough.

Action: Refer to rheumatology – to a dedicated Early Inflammatory Back Pain Clinic, if available.

Transplantation

David Talbot and Chas Newstead

In any transplant patient:

1 Skin ulcers or lumps could be neoplastic.

2 Unexplained enlarged glands – think of lymphoma.

3 Acute febrile illness without obvious signs may be infection by unusual organisms.

In a patient with a kidney transplant:

4 Sudden weight change is due to a change in fluid balance.

5 Temperature and flu-like symptoms may indicate graft rejection.

6 Pain and tenderness of the graft can be pyelonephritis, obstruction or graft rejection.

In a patient with a liver transplant:

7 Temperature, rigors and sometimes dark urine signal infective cholangitis or graft necrosis.

8 Intractable itch – think of chronic rejection.

9 A recurrence of ascites indicates portal hypertension usually from a thrombosed portal vein.

In a patient with a heart transplant:

10 Recurrence of angina or cardiac failure suggests chronic rejection.

In a patient with a lung transplant:

11 Gradual deterioration in exercise tolerance may be due to obliterative bronchiolitis.

NOTES

GENERAL

1 Skin malignancy

Skin lumps or non-healing ulcers in transplant patients on long-term immunosuppression are usually either viral or neoplastic. Viral lesions are common and can be treated topically by liquid nitrogen. Reduction in immunosuppression or treatment with isoretinoin is also sometimes possible. Due to the increased risk of skin malignancy, all transplant recipients are warned of the dangers of ultraviolet exposure. This should be reinforced at every opportunity and patients should report any new lesions. In Australia, the chances of a transplant recipient having had a squamous cell cancer by the time they get to 15 years post transplant is 80%.

Action: Urgently refer suspicious skin lesions to dermatology.

2 Post-transplant lymphoma

Post-transplant lymphoma is rare but carries a high mortality. In most cases, it is caused by the combination of immunosuppression and an infective agent (usually Epstein–Barr virus). Patients with unexplained fever or lymphadenopathy may have post-transplant lympho-proliferative disease. Early referral is important.

Action: Examine lymph nodes and refer urgently to the transplant team.

3 Atypical infection

Infections from esoteric organisms are now less common than they were. This is partly because of refinement in immunosuppression and the increased use of the prophylactic antimicrobial co-trimoxazole. However, the doctor should always beware of the patient who looks sick but has relatively minor signs. Such is the case with early *Pneumocystis* pneumonia or

Aspergillus infections. Antibiotic therapy needs to be selected with care in these patients because of drug interactions.

Action: Refer immediately to the transplant team.

KIDNEY TRANSPLANT

4 Weight change

Changes in weight reflect changes in fluid balance. Fluid loss can occur in gastroenteritis, leading quickly to dehydration and graft failure. Adequate fluid intake at such a time is important.

Weight increase over time is an indicator of fluid retention from graft failure. Sometimes the patient may know this but they hope to put off a return to dialysis as long as possible. In this case, fluid retention may be associated with pulmonary oedema, which can be life-threatening.

Action: Ensure adequate fluid intake during gastroenteritis. Refer to the transplant team, urgently if weight changes are rapid.

5 Graft rejection

Fever and flulike symptoms are potentially serious symptoms. Infection from viruses is common and usually self-limiting, but CMV infection can be serious in the early phase. Bacterial urinary infection can be occult and should be looked for. Antibiotics should be used after culture, though care needs to be exercised due to drug interactions with immunosuppressive drugs. These symptoms can also indicate graft rejection, particularly if the patient has not been taking immunosuppressive medications. If these symptoms are due to rejection, they are always associated with poor function (poor urine output and deranged renal function) and sometimes tenderness of the graft.

Action: If cause of fever is not obvious, refer urgently to the transplant team – immediately if there are signs of graft rejection.

6 Graft rejection/infarction

Unless there is a specific history of physical exercise or trauma to the kidney, pain and tenderness of a graft are ominous symptoms. Occasionally, the cause is UTI but more usually, there is acute rejection or venous infarction of the graft.

Action: Refer immediately to the transplant team.

LIVER

7 Infective cholangitis

Following transplant, the bile duct can occasionally narrow down at the site of the anastomosis. With the resulting biliary stasis, stones tend to form above the stenosis. This combination leads to episodes of cholangitis with jaundice. Temperature, rigors and sometimes dark urine may be present. This condition is also occasionally seen when a duct-to-bowel anastomosis has been created, and then the cholangitis is due to the reflux of bowel organisms into the biliary tree.

Temperature and rigors can also occur if the blood supply to the liver is blocked, such as with hepatic artery thrombosis, causing liver infarction. This is often asymptomatic but presents if the infarcted portion becomes infected.

Action: Refer immediately to the transplant team.

8 Chronic rejection

Liver transplant recipients with intractable itch usually have chronic rejection. The symptom is caused by build-up of bile salts in the skin. Typically, LFTs are abnormal and the itch responds poorly to medication.

Action: Refer to the transplant clinic.

9 Portal vein thrombosis

After liver transplant, the portal venous pressure, which is usually elevated before transplant for chronic liver disease, is near normal. If the patient subsequently develops evidence of portal hypertension such as variceal haemorrhage or ascites, portal vein thrombosis is likely.

Action: For GI haemorrhage, refer immediately to the emergency department. For ascites, refer non-urgently to the transplant team.

HEART

10 Chronic rejection

Chronic rejection of any transplanted organ usually starts with thickening of the vessel wall (intima). In the kidney, this leads to dependent ischaemia producing glomerulosclerosis, and in the liver, the bile ducts 'vanish'. In the heart, angina or cardiac failure is produced.

Action: Refer urgently to the transplant clinic.

LUNG

11 Obliterative bronchiolitis

Chronic rejection in the lung occurs by obliteration of the airways and vascular atherosclerosis. This presents as a gradual deterioration in exercise tolerance. Manipulation of immunosuppression by the specialist unit can offer some hope but once established the process is non-reversible.

Action: Refer to the transplant clinic.

Upper GI surgery

Michael Griffin and Nick Hayes

1 New onset of persistent dyspepsia warrants investigation, whatever the patient's age.

2 Progressive dysphagia demands exclusion of upper GI malignancy.

3 Regurgitation, as opposed to vomiting, suggests oesophageal stricture.

4 Do not forget upper GI causes of chest pain.

5 Nocturnal cough could be caused by aspiration episodes.

6 Coughing and spluttering on swallowing liquids may herald malignancy.

7 Rebound of upper GI symptoms after stopping PPIs – think of malignancy unmasked.

8 Obstructive jaundice frequently justifies more urgent referral, even when a benign aetiology is suspected.

NOTES

1 Dyspepsia

Dyspepsia is epigastric pain associated with eating. New onset of persistent dyspepsia (lasting over 2 weeks), in adults of any age, warrants investigation. The alarm symptoms (and signs) used in '2-week rule' guidelines to recommend prompt referral for endoscopy often relate to advanced disease, much of which is incurable. Endoscopic assessment of uncomplicated dyspepsia is more likely to pick up curable lesions. Benign disease can be diagnosed correctly to rationalise treatment, and malignancy can be detected early. To this end, it is worth assuming that there is no difference between symptoms of benign and malignant disease in the early stages.

Action: Refer for endoscopy.

2 Dysphagia

Progressive dysphagia is a cardinal symptom of upper GI malignancy and this diagnosis should always be excluded, particularly if associated with weight loss. Malignancy should be considered irrespective of the patient's age.

Action: Refer urgently using local direct access endoscopy or 2-week cancer proformas if available.

3 Oesophageal obstruction

Patients who complain of 'vomiting' might, on closer questioning, be describing effortless regurgitation. This symptom can signify an oesophageal obstructive process, such as stricture, cancer or achalasia. Patients should be asked whether their regurgitation occurs with or without retching to discriminate between these two symptoms. Barium studies are helpful in diagnosis.

Action: Refer urgently for endoscopy.

4 Upper GI causes of chest pain

Chest pain can be caused by a range of upper GI problems. Chest pain on swallowing, particularly with hot liquids (odynophagia), is often seen with erosive oesophagitis, and occasionally with cancer. The pain of heartburn is commonly recognised due to its association with meals, alcohol and posture. The discomfort of oesophageal spasm, however, is more easily confused with that of angina pectoris and is often precipitated by anxiety and, confusingly, may be relieved by nitrates. Contrast studies, using a semi-solid agent in addition to liquid barium, are helpful in diagnosis.

The rare condition of spontaneous oesophageal perforation (Boerhaave's syndrome) is usually diagnosed late after a differential of MI, pulmonary embolism or perforated peptic ulcer has been considered. The history is usually of severe thoracic pain following forceful, often prolonged, vomiting. A non-ionic contrast swallow either with conventional or CT imaging is the definitive investigation in the emergency unit.

Action: Refer for endoscopy. If considering Boerhaave's syndrome, refer immediately to upper GI surgery.

5 Reflux with aspiration

Nocturnal cough is frequently associated with cardiorespiratory disease but might be due to postural gastro-oesophageal reflux with aspiration episodes. Nocturnal aspiration is rarely controlled by medical therapy alone, and warrants referral for consideration of surgical intervention.

Action: Refer to upper GI surgery.

6 Aerodigestive fistula and recurrent laryngeal nerve palsy

Coughing or spluttering on swallowing, particularly when associated with dysphagia, indicates a patient at high risk of inhalation pneumonia. The mechanism may be bulbar incoordination, but may also be a recurrent laryngeal nerve palsy, or an aerodigestive fistula. The last two conditions are strongly associated with advanced malignancy. Endoscopy is useful, but a carefully conducted dilute barium swallow is more likely to show the anatomical abnormality. Non-ionic contrast should be avoided as it can cause severe pneumonitis if inhaled.

Action: Refer urgently to upper GI surgery.

7 Masking of upper GI malignancy by PPIs

PPIs can improve the symptoms of early malignancy as effectively as for benign ulceration and reflux processes. Symptom rebound after cessation of PPIs mandates investigation if it has not yet been done. In addition, 'normal' results following upper GI investigation must be interpreted cautiously if they were conducted while patients were taking acid suppression therapy.

Action: Arrange endoscopy when the patient has been off acid suppression therapy for 4 weeks.

8 Biliary colic with jaundice

Patients with symptoms of biliary colic ought to be referred with greater urgency if jaundice, however transient, has complicated the pain. The individual might have passed a stone via the common duct or indeed might still harbour a stone within the duct. These patients are at risk of acute pancreatitis and cholangitis and so should not be referred along a 'routine gallstones' pathway.

Action: Look for evidence of common duct dilatation on ultrasound reports of patients with gallstones. Refer more promptly any patient with a history of jaundice or common bile duct dilatation.

Urology

Jeremy Crew and Bernard Bochner

1 A boy with a painful scrotum can lose a testicle within hours.

2 Nocturnal enuresis in a man over 50 years may precede renal failure.

3 A prolonged, painful erection can end in impotency.

4 Haematuria always requires exclusion of malignancy.

5 Loin pain, fever and malaise in an insulin-dependent diabetic could represent life-threatening emphysematous pyelonephritis.

6 Renal colic with fever may signify an infected obstructed kidney.

7 Blood at the urethral meatus in a pelvic trauma victim – think of posterior urethral injury.

8 Always consider bladder rupture in blunt, lower abdominal injury.

NOTES

1 Testicular torsion

The child or neonate presenting with acute scrotal pain is a true urological emergency. Testicular torsion may be present, which can cause irreversible testicular damage within 6 h of the onset of symptoms. While the differential diagnosis also includes epididymitis, trauma, tumour and inguinal hernia, torsion should always be considered first and promptly ruled out. Surgical detorsion within 6 h will usually result in normal testicular function.

Action: Refer immediately to paediatric urology for emergency surgery.

2 Chronic urinary retention

Benign prostatic hyperplasia is common in men over 50 years. This can lead to symptoms of bladder outlet obstruction and chronic retention. The bladder pressure may remain high in chronic retention and can be transmitted to the upper tracts leading to renal impairment. Nocturnal enuresis in an adult is highly suggestive of chronic retention.

Action: Examine for a distended bladder. If a full bladder is palpable, measure renal function immediately. If it is deranged, perform urethral catheterisation without delay. Monitor urine output following catheterisation (diuresis may occur). Admission and IV rehydration may be necessary. If bladder is not distended, do urinalysis to exclude UTI and abdominal X-ray to exclude bladder calculi.

3 Priapism

Priaprism is persistent penile erection without sexual desire. Obstruction of the cavernosal venous system prevents the outflow of blood from the corpus cavernosum. Hypoxia of the penile tissues can lead to irreversible fibrosis and impotency. Pain and difficultly voiding are common associated symptoms.

Painful erections signify that tissue hypoxia and damage are present. Etiologies include drugs (intracavernosal injection therapy, psychotropics, antihypertensives, anticoagulants), sickle cell disease or trait, neoplasia, and trauma. Some cases are idiopathic.

Action: Relieve pain – narcotics may be useful. In sickle cell patients, give oxygen and ensure hydration. In the acute state, refer immediately to urology.

4 Urological malignancy

Microscopic or gross blood in the urine may be the presenting feature of a life-threatening urothelial cancer or tumour of the renal parenchyma (renal cell cancer). The differential diagnosis for haematuria includes tumour, urinary calculi, infection, medical renal disease, benign prostatic hypertrophy and trauma. Because of the potential for a malignant cause, haematuria (microscopic or gross) should never be ignored and must be worked up regardless of its severity or intermittency. Investigation includes an upper tract imaging evaluation and cystoscopy.

Action: Refer urgently to urology.

5 Emphysematous pyelonephritis

Emphysematous pyelonephritis is a severe, rare complication of acute pyelonephritis caused by glucose-fermenting bacteria (typically *Escherichia coli*) that produce gas within the renal parenchyma. It is most frequently seen in poorly controlled, insulin-dependent diabetics or patients with obstructing ureteral or renal pelvic stones. The symptoms include loin pain, fever and malaise. Prompt diagnosis is critical so that emergency therapy can be instituted. This involves immediate IV antibiotics, imaging and possible nephrectomy. Emphysematous pyelonephritis carries up to 50% mortality.

Action: Refer immediately to urology.

6 Infected obstructed kidney

Renal and ureteric colic present classically with symptoms of severe loin pain radiating towards the groin. Occasionally, though, there may be a superadded urinary infection. The combination of infection and high-pressure ureteric obstruction is potentially fatal through Gram-negative septicemia. Whenever a diagnosis of ureteric colic has been made, therefore, UTI should be excluded. Ongoing or worsening urinary sepsis (fever, tachycardia, hypotension, raised white cell count) demands urgent surgery to relieve the obstruction. In adults, also consider the differential of a leaking abdominal aortic aneurysm.

Action: Check temperature and dipstick urine. If pyrexia is present, or dipstick is positive for nitrites, start high-dose IV antibiotics and refer immediately to urology.

7 Posterior urethral injury

Pelvic fractures, particularly those that involve the pubic ramus, may be associated with a posterior urethral injury. The injury more commonly affects men. Over 80% of patients present with blood at the urethral meatus. Digital rectal examination will frequently identify a 'high-riding' prostate located in a more superior position in the pelvis. Up to 20% of posterior urethral injuries will have an associated rupture of the bladder.

Action: Peform a digital rectal examination to check for prostate position. Do not insert a urethral catheter until a retrograde urethrogram has confirmed urethral integrity. If extravasation is noted, insert a suprapubic catheter instead.

8 Ruptured bladder

Bladder rupture should always be considered where there is a history of blunt lower abdominal injury, such as deceleration road traffic accident. The symptoms are often non-specific and may initially be mild. Intraperitoneal rupture requires surgical closure. Extraperitoneal rupture can be managed conservatively unless the patient's condition deteriorates.

Action: Arrange immediate cystography to confirm the diagnosis.

Vascular surgery

Gerard Stansby, Shervanthi Homer-Vanniasinkam and Mohan Adiseshiah

1 Sudden onset of severe abdominal pain, back pain or 'renal colic' in a patient over 60 years – think of abdominal aortic aneurysm rupture.

2 Sudden onset of weakness and numbness in the leg may not be stroke – exclude acute lower limb ischaemia.

3 Severe pain in the dorsum of the foot could mean critical ischaemia.

4 An elderly patient with severe, generalised abdominal pain and diarrhoea – consider mesenteric ischaemia.

5 Transient neurological deficit – stroke may be prevented.

6 Calf pain on walking is a portent of coronary artery disease.

7 Ipsilateral headache in a patient who has recently had carotid endarterectomy could be life-threatening.

8 Pyrexia in a patient with a previous vascular graft – consider graft infection.

9 Bleeding from a varicose vein can lead to exsanguination.

10 A leg ulcer that fails to heal despite treatment may be malignant.

NOTES

1 Ruptured abdominal aortic aneurysm (AAA)

A ruptured AAA is an abdominal catastrophe and the patient requires emergency surgery to have a chance of survival. It is one of the commonest causes of death in males over 60 years. Back or loin pain can be the first sign of leak or impending rupture. Pain may radiate into the groin and there may be blood in the urine because of haematoma around the kidney and ureter – misdiagnosis as renal colic is not uncommon. Sweating, pallor and signs of shock may be present. Frequently the patient recovers from an initial episode and appears quite well for a while before relapsing. Ultrasound or computed tomography (CT) will confirm the diagnosis.

Action: Always consider AAA in the differential of back, loin or abdominal pain. Palpate for a tender, pulsatile mass. Arrange imaging if this will not delay referral. Refer immediately to vascular surgery.

2 Acute lower limb ischaemia

Sudden onset of weakness and numbness in the leg may be due to acute ischaemia from an embolus or thrombosis in one of the major limb arteries such as the common femoral artery. Although pain is one of the well-known features of acute limb ischaemia (pain, pallor, pulselessness, paraesthesia and paralysis), paradoxically more severe ischaemia may be less painful because of nerve involvement. In these cases, the leg becomes more numb than painful. Such cases are sometimes misdiagnosed as stroke. Acute ischaemia of the leg is a true surgical emergency since irreversible ischaemia can occur after just 4–6 h. Unfortunately, particularly in debilitated, bedridden patients, the diagnosis is often not made until late skin changes occur. Then, amputation is all that can be done.

Action: Examine the legs for signs of acute ischaemia, including feeling for peripheral pulses. Refer immediately to vascular surgery.

3 Critical limb ischaemia

Foot pain at rest is an ominous feature of critical ischaemia – the limb is in peril. Ischaemic rest pain is localised to the forefoot (transmetatarsal) and should be differentiated from benign, nocturnal, calf muscle cramps, which are common in elderly patients. The patient may be awakened by ischaemic rest pain, or may be unable to sleep because of it. The limb is hung over the edge of the bed in an attempt to gain relief. The foot assumes a crimson hue ('sunset foot'). There may be trophic changes in the foot (muscle wasting, thickened nails, thin skin, hair loss in the limb). Simple friction between adjacent toes results in 'kissing ulcers' in the interdigital clefts. Revascularisation or amputation may be needed.

Action: Refer urgently to vascular surgery.

4 Mesenteric ischaemia

Occlusion of the mesenteric circulation is not commonly seen, but can be catastrophic if the diagnosis is missed. It can present acutely, due to mesenteric thromboembolism: an elderly patient with severe abdominal pain out of proportion to the physical findings, possibly with nausea and diarrhoea, which may be bloody. Chronically, the diagnosis is harder to make and it is common for a patient to have 'done the rounds' before reaching a vascular surgeon. Patients are usually females who report postprandial abdominal pain, weight loss and 'food fear'. The differential here includes malignancy and chronic pancreatitis.

Action: Refer to vascular surgery, immediately in acute cases.

5 TIA

TIAs are brief episodes (< 24 h) of focal loss of brain function due to ischaemia. They are localised to a particular arterial territory (internal carotid artery or vertebrobasilar).

Carotid artery TIAs cause amaurosis fugax (sudden, transient loss of vision in one eye only) as well as transient dysarthria, weakness or paraesthesia of a limb, facial weakness or aphasia. These are usually due to carotid stenosis, which is the only curable condition in the field of stroke disease. Untreated, the patient is at risk of blindness or massive cortical infarct. Carotid endarterectomy has clear benefit in preventing stroke.

Action: Perform a neurological and cardiovascular examination. Refer urgently for carotid Dopplers and then to vascular surgery (or directly to a specialist TIA clinic). Commence aspirin, or alternative antiplatelet therapy, if no contraindications. Address vascular risk factors.

6 Intermittent claudication

In itself, calf pain on walking (intermittent claudication) is not sinister for the limb – only around 10% of claudicating limbs will develop critical or acute ischaemia. However, it is a sad fact that half of these patients will be dead within 5 years from coronary artery disease. The symptom is therefore a major pointer to this condition.

Action: Carry out a thorough cardiovascular history and examination and do an ECG. Assess vascular risk factors and treat these aggressively. Refer to cardiology if ischaemic heart disease is suspected.

7 Reperfusion syndrome

In the days following carotid endarterectomy, the patient is usually at home. If the patient complains of severe hemicranial headache, especially on the side of the carotid endarterectomy, the possibility of reperfusion syndrome should be borne in mind. This is a condition of impaired cerebrovascular autoregulation, and is a rare complication of endarterectomy. Untreated, it could lead to cerebral haemorrhage and stroke, sometimes fatally. Management involves urgent readmission, CT scanning and control of the blood pressure.

Action: Refer immediately to vascular surgery.

8 Infected vascular graft

Prosthetic vascular grafts may become infected at any time after implantation – even several years. Organisms may lie dormant from the time of the original operation, or may enter following bacteraemia due to dental extraction or catheterisation. Any pyrexia without obvious cause in a patient with a prior vascular graft should therefore be considered as a possible sign of a graft infection. Aortic graft infection has a mortality of approximately 50% and infection of a graft in the leg has an amputation rate of 50%. Usually graft removal is needed.

Action: Carry out standard investigations for pyrexia of unknown origin. Arrange CT of graft and labelled white cell isotope scan. Refer urgently to vascular surgery.

9 Varicose vein bleed

Varicose veins are usually regarded as relatively innocuous. However, large varicosities can bleed torrentially if there is a break in the overlying skin. A typical patient would be an elderly female with thin, atrophic skin. A minor injury, even scratching, can open the vein leading to painless bleeding. This may go unnoticed, perhaps when the patient is asleep in a chair. In such circumstances, death from exsanguination can occur.

Action: Apply digital pressure and elevate leg to control bleeding. Refer urgently to vascular surgery.

10 Marjolin's ulcer

If a venous ulcer fails to improve despite appropriate treatment with elevation and compression bandaging, malignant transformation in the ulcer may have occurred. This is termed a Marjolin's ulcer.

Action: Refer urgently to vascular surgery or dermatology.

Index

abdominal malignancy 36
abdominal symptoms,
    non-GI causes of 38
abdominal aortic aneurysm (AAA),
    ruptured 159
acoustic neuroma 32
acute closed-angle glaucoma
    (ACAG) 94
Addison's disease 27, 69
    and thyroid hormone
        replacement 27–28
Addisonian crisis 141
AIDS 22
airway burn 120
alcohol withdrawl, acute 128
allergic bronchopulmonary
        aspergillosis (ABPA) 66–67
altered vaginal discharge 40
anaemia 52
    iron deficiency 35–36
anastomotic leak 37–38
angio-oedema 22–23
    acquired 65
    hereditary (HAE) 64–65
ankylosing spondylitis 143
anogenital
    ulcers 41
    warts 41
anorexia 36
    nervosa 127
antineutrophil cytoplasmic
        antibodies (ANCAs) 65
antiphospholipid syndrome 66
anxiety disorders 128
aortic
    coarctation 12, 110

stenosis 11
    symptoms 11
    transection 14
appendicitis, acute 118
arrhythmia 6, 12
    atrial fibrillation 9
    brady 6
    tachy 6
arrhythmic syncope 6, 110
ascites 55
asthma
    aspirin-sensitive asthma
        137–138
    uncontrolled 136
atrial fibrillation 9
    treatment 9
atypical infection 145–146

back pain, acute
    medical causes of 108
bacterial meningitis 76
Baker's cyst, ruptured 142
Bell's palsy 77, 102
biliary
    atresia 111
    colic
        with jaundice 152
bipolar disorder 127
bladder, ruptured 156–157
bleeding
    rectal 35
    upper GI 36–37
    varices 56
Boerhaave's syndrome 151
brain tumour 113
breast asymmetry 3